Instant Pot Mediterranean Diet Cookbook

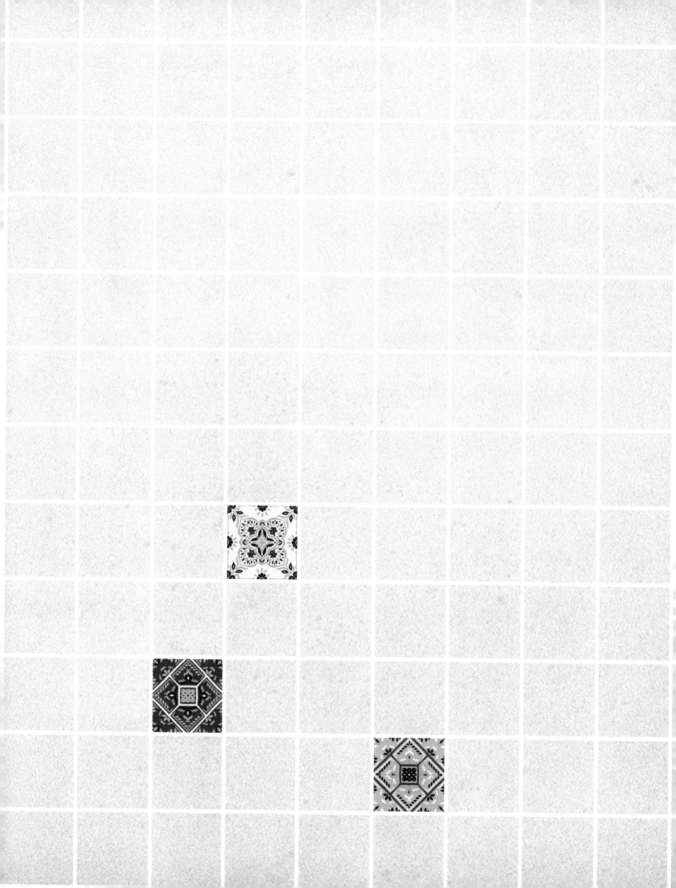

INSTANT POT MEDITERRANEAN DIET COOKBOOK

75 QUICK MEALS FOR A HEALTHY LIFESTYLE

Abbie Gellman, MS, RD, CDN

ROCKRIDGE
PRESS

For general information on our other products and services or to obtain technical support, please contact our Customer Care Department within the United States at (866) 744-2665, or outside the United States at (510) 253-0500.

Rockridge Press publishes its books in a variety of electronic and print formats. Some content that appears in print may not be available in electronic books, and vice versa.

These recipes were previously published in *Mediterranean Pressure Cooking*.

Cover Designer: Amanda Kirk
Interior Designer: Scott Wooledge
Art Producer: Alyssa Williams
Editor: Sierra Machado
Production Editor: Ruth Sakata Corley
Production Manager: Martin Worthington

Photography © 2022 Darren Muir, Food styling by Yolanda Muir, cover and pp. vi, x, 12, 27, 45, 50, 84, 92, 118, 132; © Andrew Purcell, pp. viii, 22, 34, 60, 74, 77, 96, 110, 123, 143. Tile Illustrations © AndrewPixel/Creative Market

Paperback ISBN: 978-1-63878-362-6
eBook ISBN: 978-1-63878-522-4
R0

*Thanks to all of you who have
picked up this book and taken it into the
kitchen—cooking, trying new
things, and getting your hands dirty.*

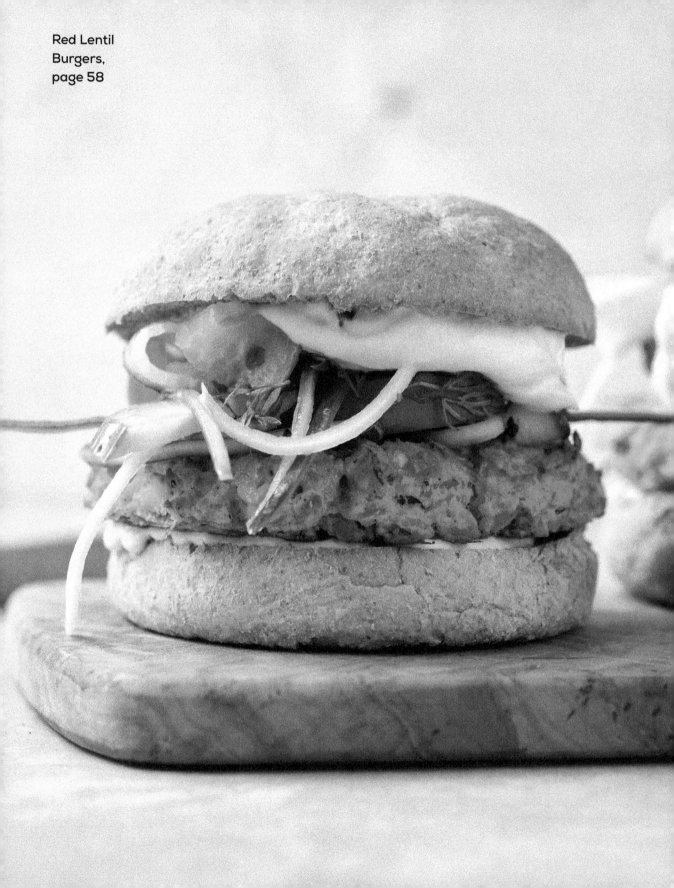

Red Lentil
Burgers,
page 58

CONTENTS

Introduction ix

CHAPTER ONE: **MEDITERRANEAN COOKING WITH THE INSTANT POT** 1

CHAPTER TWO: **THE MEDITERRANEAN KITCHEN** 13

CHAPTER THREE: **BREAKFAST** 23

CHAPTER FOUR: **VEGETABLES AND SIDES** 35

CHAPTER FIVE: **MEATLESS MAINS** 51

CHAPTER SIX: **SEAFOOD** 75

CHAPTER SEVEN: **POULTRY AND MEAT** 93

CHAPTER EIGHT: **DESSERT** 119

CHAPTER NINE: **SAUCES AND STAPLES** 133

Instant Pot Cooking Charts . . . 146

Measurement Conversions . . . 152

Reference 154

Index 155

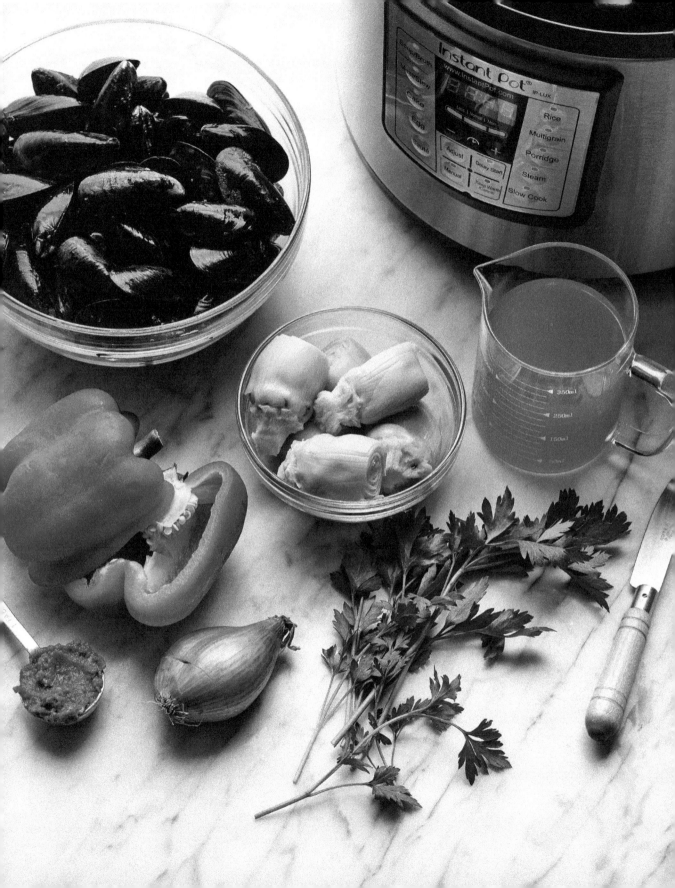

INTRODUCTION

I love food. As a chef and registered dietitian, I have a passion for making food that is both healthy and delicious. It is this tenet—along with the idea that food should bring joy and help foster community—that I keep in mind when I create recipes and cook to feed and nourish myself and others.

The Mediterranean diet is a relatively simple style of eating and cooking that I have followed for years. It focuses on using fresh, whole foods—such as fruits, vegetables, beans, and lean protein—and brings an abundance of flavor from a variety of herbs and spices. It is straightforward recipes with these ingredients that empower the readers and viewers of my videos and website, ChefAbbieGellman.com.

I also love my Instant Pot and have found it to be an invaluable appliance, especially when I am following a Mediterranean diet. Its overall convenience and adaptability have made it a workhorse in many a modern kitchen. My favorite part is that the Instant Pot makes healthy cooking easy, tasty, and—best of all—efficient!

As you make your way through this book, there are guidelines and general information regarding the Mediterranean diet and lifestyle. This book also includes information about the Instant Pot—how to use it, safety and trouble-shooting tips, and helpful tools and accessories.

Finally, there are dozens of easy, delicious, and healthy Mediterranean diet recipes made with accessible ingredients that can be found at your local grocery store or, in some cases, ordered online. These recipes focus on whole foods, and many can be enjoyed even if you have dietary restrictions, such as dairy-free or gluten-free. Each recipe includes tips that provide helpful information, swap ideas, shortcuts, or freezing tips, as well as nutritional information.

Thanks for joining me in the Mediterranean kitchen with your Instant Pot. I hope you love these recipes and the Mediterranean diet as much as I do and that this book becomes an integral part of your kitchen and cooking experience.

IX

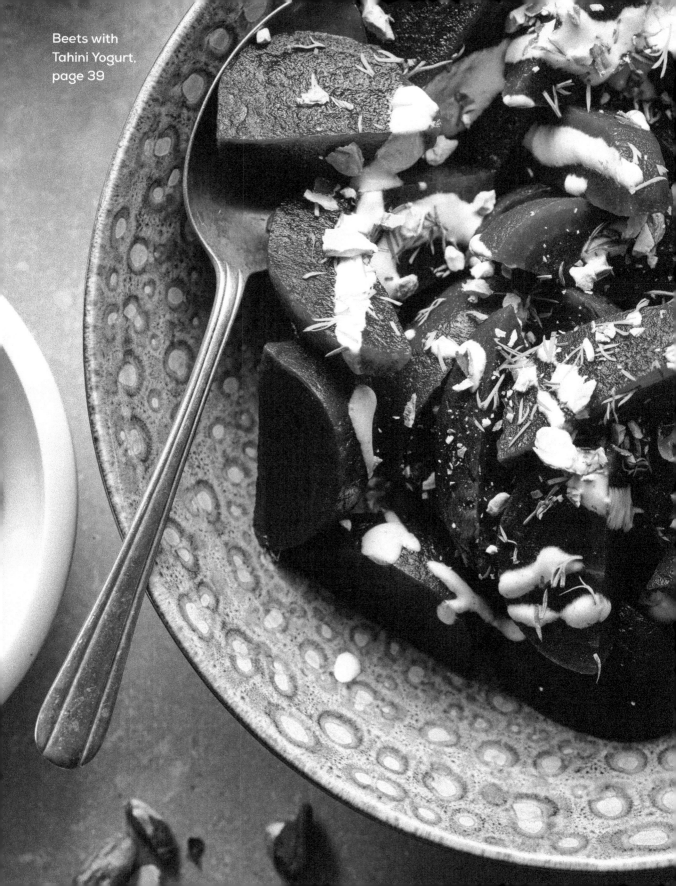

Beets with
Tahini Yogurt,
page 39

CHAPTER ONE

MEDITERRANEAN COOKING WITH THE INSTANT POT

EATING THE MEDITERRANEAN WAY

The Mediterranean diet, ranked as the number one best diet overall and the number one best plant-based diet by *U.S. News & World Report* in 2019 and 2020, is relatively simple in nature. It places an emphasis on eating a variety of whole foods—such as vegetables, whole grains, nuts, and lean protein—and is primarily plant-based. This means that there is a larger emphasis placed on the consumption of plant-based foods than animal-based foods.

Although some diets are extremely rigid, the Mediterranean diet instead provides simple guidelines for improving your eating habits without leaving you feeling deprived or restricted. It is more of a lifestyle and way of thinking that extends beyond just food. On a Mediterranean diet, we can achieve health and wellness with a long-term, holistic view of eating, moving, and living that helps prevent the onset of chronic disease and promote longevity.

Here are five main tenets of the Mediterranean diet and lifestyle.

■ Health without Sacrifice

The Mediterranean diet focuses on nourishing, nutritious ingredients without sacrificing flavor. There are no rules about certain foods being "off limits" or "forbidden." Instead, the emphasis is on moderation.

■ Quality Over Quantity

The Mediterranean diet is a plant-based approach to eating centered on an abundance of fresh whole foods, ranging from fruits and vegetables to nuts and legumes and lean animal proteins like dairy and seafood. It prioritizes choosing quality over quantity, so, in general, the portion sizes may be smaller than the standard American or Western diet, but the quality of the food will shine through and leave you satisfied.

■ Cultivating Community

The pleasures of cooking and enjoying a meal among family and friends go hand in hand. The Mediterranean diet and lifestyle are not only about food but also about community, sharing meals with others, and spending time together. Part of cultivating community also includes slowing down to truly enjoy meals and appreciating indulgences like red wine in moderation.

■ Preserving Culture and Tradition

The Mediterranean diet is about not only ingredients and recipes but also people, their lives, and where they live. It is steeped in tradition, highlighting flavors and foods that have been passed down through generations as a way of preserving memories and culture.

■ Staying Active

Staying physically active and moving is crucial for optimal health and wellness. All physical movement counts, from doing yoga to taking a walk or going for a leisurely swim. Exercise and activity do not have to be competitive or strenuous; the point is to move your body every day.

PARADISE MEETS THE POT

The modern Instant Pot is a great way to get you started on the Mediterranean diet. Here are my top reasons why this dynamic duo can give you a push in the right direction.

Healthy meals with less effort: Many conventional cooking methods require constant supervision or more hands-on cooking time in addition to the up-front prep time. The Instant Pot allows you to skip that and still have delicious, healthy meals regularly. The majority of recipes in this book are made fully in the Instant Pot, so once all the ingredients are sealed in the pot, you simply set it and walk away.

Redefines "fast food": Many stews, braises, and other dishes that typically take a long time to cook can be made quickly in the Instant Pot. Those of us who always feel like we're short on time or simply don't want to spend hours in the kitchen can make a wide variety of healthy, delicious homemade meals without limitations.

More flavorful meals: Instant Pot cooking creates a closed environment so flavor molecules cannot escape the way they might in a conventional cooking method. A reduced amount of added liquid in an Instant Pot recipe is also a means to concentrate flavor. In the case of animal proteins—such as whole chickens or cuts of meat—the natural juices stay put, resulting in juicy, flavorful meat and poultry.

Saves you money: In many instances, Instant Pots take less time to cook food compared to other conventional methods and do not use a stovetop or oven. Pressure cookers, including Instant Pots, use 50 to 75 percent less energy, according to the American Council for an Energy-Efficient Economy. Shortened cooking times and less energy use translate to lower energy bills and more money in your pocket. In addition, there are many foods, such as dried beans and legumes, that are cheaper than their canned counterparts and are used frequently in the Mediterranean diet.

HOW THE INSTANT POT WORKS

Instant Pots function based on one overarching principle: that the temperature of boiling liquid is higher in an enclosed, tightly sealed environment. As a result, the time it takes to boil, braise, or steam is greatly reduced.

Once the Instant Pot lid is sealed, locked in place, and turned on, steam develops and cannot escape. These trapped water molecules increase the pressure inside the Instant Pot by an average of 12 to 15 pounds per square inch (psi), or 12 to 15 pounds above normal sea level pressure, which raises the boiling point of water from 212°F to between 244°F and 250°F. Depending on the model, Instant Pots may have different setting options. A "low" setting of about 5 to 10 psi, or 227°F to 240°F, may be helpful for more delicate foods like puddings or coddled eggs.

Pressure cooking allows you to make healthy, flavorful dishes using whole foods in less time, with minimal cleanup, and often with less oil or added fat. And here's a bonus: Food cooked in the Instant Pot retains more nutrients than boiled food since there's less liquid for vitamins and minerals to leech out into!

THE MEDITERRANEAN REGION

The Mediterranean region, encompassing more than 20 countries, is diverse from both a cultural and culinary point of view. There's no singular diet eaten by all the countries that border the Mediterranean Sea. Instead of specific dishes, the Mediterranean diet focuses on the abundance of healthy foods available in countries across the region. Inspiration for the recipes in this cookbook mainly comes from the following Mediterranean countries.

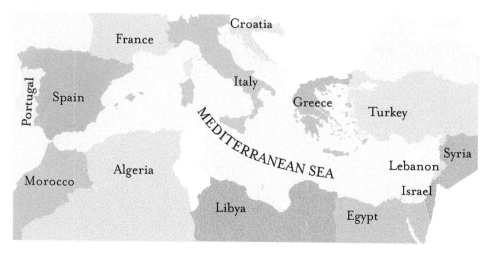

INSTANT POT PARTS AND SETTINGS

Instant Pots are available in a range of prices and sizes, suitable to meet most budget and batch-cooking needs. The average size you'll find most often is a 6-quart Instant Pot, which easily makes recipes with four to six servings. For some ingredients, such as beans, legumes, and grains, the 6-quart size can easily batch-cook a pound of each.

Smaller 3-quart Instant Pots are also widely available. These take up less counter space, but you will be limited in the amount of food that you can cook at one time. For those who like to cook large batches or regularly have more mouths to feed, 8-quart Instant Pots are a good choice. For the purposes of this cookbook, all recipes were developed and tested using a 6-quart Instant Pot.

There are a variety of universal settings and instructions you'll encounter when cooking with Instant Pots. The following list provides additional information regarding the ones you will see in this cookbook:

Sauté/Brown: Sautéing or browning some foods like meat and poultry or aromatics, such as onions and garlic, adds depth and flavor to the finished dish. This is not a pressure setting, so take care to not close the locking lid when using it.

Adding liquid: Liquid is integral to the pressure-cooking process since it essentially becomes the steam that creates pressure and cooks the food. Sufficient liquid is required if you want the Instant Pot to work properly.

Locking the lid: The way in which your lid locks in place depends on the model, so be sure to follow the manufacturer's instructions. Generally speaking, you line up a specific part of the lid with a precise area on the pot and twist the lid into place. There is also a steam valve that should be set to sealed, although on some models this is automatically done.

High pressure: Generally, the high-pressure setting registers at roughly 12 to 15 psi. The majority of recipes use the high-pressure setting since it is most efficient. Please note that once you hit the high-pressure button on the Instant Pot, it takes roughly 10 minutes to get up to pressure. This means that the timer does not activate until that happens. As such, all high-pressure recipes in this cookbook account for an additional 10 minutes in the "total time."

Low pressure: Generally, the low-pressure setting registers at roughly 10 psi. The recipes that use low pressure usually require gentler cooking, such as fish, puddings, and certain egg dishes. Please note that once you hit the low-pressure button on the Instant Pot, it takes roughly 5 minutes to get up to pressure. This means that the timer does not activate until that happens. As such, all low-pressure recipes in this cookbook account for an additional 5 minutes in the "total time."

Quick release: Quick release is used when you want to stop the cooking process immediately or do not need to finish the recipe gently. To quick release, you release the steam valve from sealed to venting, which quickly and safely releases the steam that has built up in the Instant Pot.

Natural release: Natural release is used when you want to allow the pressure to drop down naturally or finish the recipe gently. In this method, you turn off the Instant Pot, the steam valve remains closed, and the food continues to cook as the pressure dissipates over time. This can take anywhere from 15 minutes to 1 hour, depending on the recipe. In some cases, you can use natural release for a certain amount of time, then finish with a quick release.

INSTANT POT SAFETY

New to the Instant Pot? No problem! As with any kitchen appliance, knowing how to safely use it is key. Luckily for us, Instant Pots are built with multiple safety features and are easier to use than ever before. The following safety tips will help you get started and keep you cooking safely and successfully.

TIP 1: Check the equipment. The rubber gasket, which is the ring of rubber that lines the cooker lid, should not be dried out or cracked. Checking to make sure the rim of the pot is clear of any dried food is also helpful to ensure that the seal cannot be broken during cooking.

TIP 2: Never "deep-fry" in your Instant Pot. Instant Pots are meant to use liquid, such as water or broth, to create steam and pressure. Large amounts of oil can be dangerous and may cause the gasket to warp at high temperatures.

TIP 3: Use enough liquid, but do not overfill the inner pot. Enough liquid is required to create steam and maintain pressure. However, take care not to fill beyond the inner pot's "max line," or the Instant Pot may spit it out when you release pressure and open the lid after cooking. This is particularly true for foods that may froth or expand during cooking, such as grains and dried beans.

TIP 4: Release pressure safely. This is especially important for quick release! Make sure your face, hands, and body are away from the vent, or you could be burned by hot steam. Once pressure is fully released, the lid should easily twist. Never try to force it open.

TIP 5: Clean and store the cooker properly. This includes the inner pot as well as the lid and gasket. Store the lid upside down in the Instant Pot versus locked in place.

TIP 6: Run an initial water test. To do this, place 3 cups of water in the Instant Pot, close the lid, turn the steam release valve to the "sealed" position, and select high pressure for 5 minutes. Once the cooking time is complete, move the steam release valve to the "venting" position and quick release the steam.

HELPFUL ACCESSORIES

You can absolutely use your Instant Pot to make delicious meals without buying any supplementary accessories. There are, however, some useful tools that may be a helpful and fun addition to your pressure cooker repertoire.

Silicone Mini Mitts: These heat-resistant mitts protect your hands from steam, and the silicone allows you to easily grip the inner pot, steam racks, or bowls and safely lift them out.

Tongs: Tongs are a very helpful tool for reaching into the pot and turning or tossing ingredients. A variety of types are available, but silicone or stainless steel generally works best.

Wire Metal Steam Rack: This should come with your Instant Pot, but you may want to purchase an extra steam rack or stackable steam racks. It has arms that are used to place foods in or lift foods out of the pot. The steam rack is often used to keep foods directly off the bottom of the inner pot. Be sure to wear heat-resistant mitts when touching the rack immediately after cooking.

Steamer Basket: This handy accessory is used to steam vegetables and is available in wire mesh, silicone, or expandable metal.

Silicone Egg Bites Mold: These stackable silicone molds allow you to make fun treats like egg bites! You can also use them for other bite-size recipes.

Ramekins: A set of 1-cup or 4-ounce ramekins is ideal for coddled eggs and individual desserts.

Loaf Pan: This is a great tool if you want to make meat loaf, quick bread, or cake recipes in your Instant Pot.

CLEANING AND CARING FOR YOUR INSTANT POT

Instant Pots are amazing appliances and a breeze to clean! Follow these tips to make sure you're keeping all the different parts clean and in tip-top shape.

Wash it out immediately. The inner pot should be removed and filled with hot, soapy water immediately after use.

Soak if necessary. The inner pot may be soaked if necessary and scrubbed as you would any other pot.

Wipe down the outside. Use a paper towel or microfiber cloth spritzed with distilled white vinegar to wipe down the outer casing of the cooker.

Clean the rim. Get a cotton swab, foam paint brush, or straw with a cotton ball or paper towel attached to the end, dip it in distilled white vinegar, then run it around the rim of the pressure cooker to clean it out.

Clean the sealing ring. This does not need to be done every time you use the Instant Pot, but the frequency may depend on how often you use the quick release function and whether or not you cook sticky or pungent foods. Detach the sealing ring from the lid, then run it through the dishwasher. Alternatively, you can pour 2 cups of distilled white vinegar and some lemon zest into the inner pot, close and seal the lid, pressure cook on low for 2 minutes, and quick release.

TIPS AND TROUBLESHOOTING

Dealing with issues that come up while using an Instant Pot is different than using conventional cooking methods. Because you cannot take off the lid "for a peek" or know what's really happening during the pressure-cooking process, you may encounter some issues after the dish is done cooking. The following is a list of common problems that may arise and solutions to help solve them.

PROBLEM: **Scorching**

SOLUTION: Scorching is often the result of not adding enough liquid. Be sure to follow the recipe and use an adequate amount of liquid.

PROBLEM: **Overcooked food**

SOLUTION: Never switch the Instant Pot to the "keep warm" setting. For quick release recipes, release the pressure immediately once the pressurized time is done. For natural release recipes, turn off the Instant Pot immediately once the pressurized time is done, then allow it to naturally release for the required amount of time as indicated in the recipe.

PROBLEM: **Uneven cooking**

SOLUTION: Follow the recipe, and prep the ingredients as directed.

PROBLEM: **Undercooked food**

SOLUTION: If you open the lid and find that the food is undercooked, simply hit the sauté button and simmer the food until cooked through. You can also transfer the contents to a stovetop pot and gently simmer there, adding liquid as needed.

PROBLEM: ## Sauce is too thin or too thick

SOLUTION: If the sauce is thinner than you like, simply hit the sauté button and simmer until it thickens to your liking. If the sauce is too thick, add more water or broth until it reaches your desired consistency.

PROBLEM: ## Cooking at high altitude

SOLUTION: At high altitudes, liquids evaporate faster and boil at lower temperatures compared to sea level. Most manufacturers include instructions regarding how to adjust cooking time. However, the general rule is to increase cooking time by 5 percent for every 1,000 feet you are located more than 2,000 feet above sea level. For example, if you are 4,000 feet above sea level and the cooking time is 30 minutes, you would increase that by 10 percent to 33 minutes. You may also have to add slightly more liquid to compensate for the additional time.

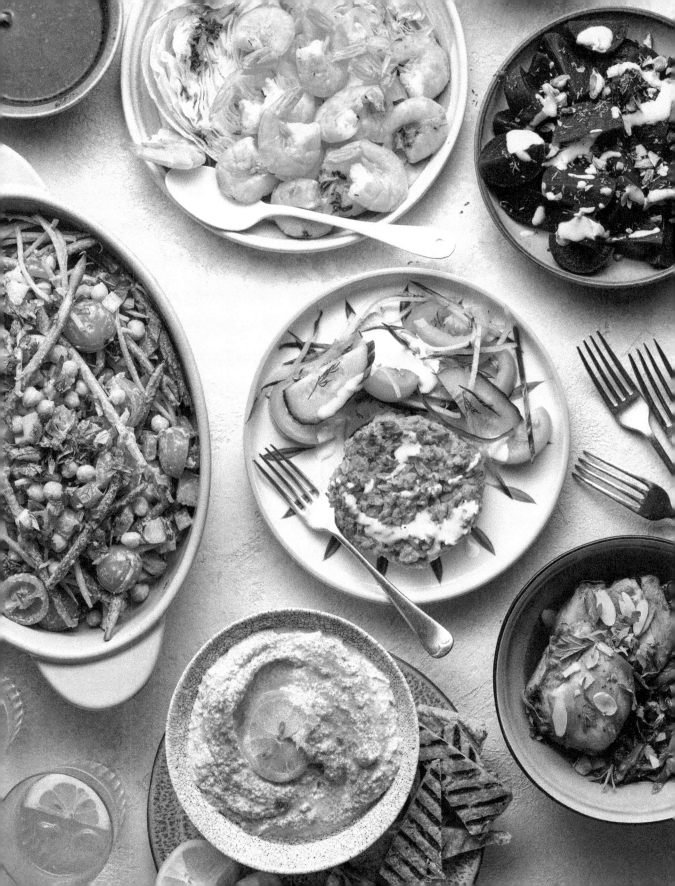

CHAPTER TWO

THE MEDITERRANEAN KITCHEN

A MEDITERRANEAN MEAL

The typical Mediterranean diet offers plenty of animal-based lean protein options, such as fish, eggs, and low-fat dairy, to name a few. It is a plant-based approach, but it is not a specifically vegan or vegetarian diet; however, you can easily take a Mediterranean approach if you follow either of those diets.

Mediterranean recipes are renowned for their simple cooking techniques and use of locally sourced whole foods. A variety of spices and herbs work together seamlessly to create flavor, texture, and healthy, delicious meals. Mediterranean meals may vary widely. Dinner could be a bowl filled with hummus and sautéed greens and vegetables topped with toasted nuts, or it could be a piece of roasted fish topped with pesto and served with braised lentils and tomatoes. As an overall lifestyle, the Mediterranean diet is easy to adhere to, with more and more people following it every year.

PLANT-BASED POWERHOUSES

The bulk of the Mediterranean diet is made up of vegetables, fruits, beans, legumes, and whole grains; these are the lifeblood of the Mediterranean kitchen. When prepared and cooked in the Instant Pot, these plant-based powerhouses shine. Beans, legumes, and grains in particular are superstars when it comes to pressure cooking.

Vegetables and Fruits

Fruits and vegetables are the workhorses of the Mediterranean diet. Full of vitamins, minerals, and antioxidants, these nutrient dynamos help power our day. Fruits and vegetables are inherently fiber-rich foods that help us feel full, support decreased blood pressure, assist with weight management, and fend off inflammation and a variety of chronic diseases. Eat a variety of fruits and vegetables every day, from berries to bananas, garlic, onion, broccoli, and cauliflower—all of these can boost your mental and physical health.

Servings: Aim to consume five to seven servings of vegetables and three or four servings of fruit daily. One serving equates to ½ cup of fruit or vegetables or 1 cup of raw leafy greens. Adding a fruit or vegetable to every meal or snack is a great way to get you there!

Instant Pot Tips: Most fruits and vegetables can be cooked in the Instant Pot. However, some are delicate and cook quickly, so many fruit and vegetable recipes use a quick release method.

Beans and Legumes

These plant-based protein sources include a variety of types, such as cannellini, kidney, and pinto beans; lentils; and soybeans. They are low in fat and high in fiber, complex carbohydrates, and protein, and they are a breeze to make in the Instant Pot from their dried state. Other key nutrients found in beans and legumes include iron, magnesium, and folate.

Servings: Aim for at least three servings of beans or legumes every week. One serving is ½ cup of cooked beans or legumes. Eating beans or legumes as a side dish or adding them to a salad or grain is an easy way to get them into your week in a delicious way.

Instant Pot Tips: Soaking beans for 8 to 24 hours prior to cooking helps cut down the total cooking time. Some people choose to soak their dried beans prior to cooking them in the Instant Pot. However, the whole point of the pressure cooker (in my opinion) is to cut down on steps and overplanning, so most of the bean recipes you find in this book do not require soaking overnight.

◼ Whole Grains and Starchy Vegetables

Whole grains and starchy vegetables are a good source of fiber, which helps slow the absorption of glucose in the blood. Packed with nutrients, these foods should be chosen over refined or processed carbohydrates whenever possible. Starchy vegetables include potatoes and sweet potatoes; whole grains include brown rice, farro, barley, oats, and whole-grain pasta.

Servings: Aim for four to six servings daily. One serving equates to ½ cup of cooked grains, 1 slice of whole-grain bread, or 1 medium sweet potato.

Instant Pot Tips: Whole grains do very well in the Instant Pot, so they are quick and delicious. However, the moisture content in the individual grains vary, so they may get tender at different times. But never fear! If you open the lid after the cooking time ends and find your whole grains a bit too "al dente," simply lock the lid back in place and leave them for a few minutes to steam.

HEALTHY ANIMAL PROTEINS

The Mediterranean diet places a heavier emphasis on fish and seafood, with smaller portions of eggs, low-fat dairy, and lean cuts of poultry and meat. Overall, you are aiming for 6 ounces of protein on a daily basis. Quick-cooking cuts of seafood, meat, and poultry that are typically cooked on the stove or grill—such as sole, filet mignon, and chicken cutlets—are generally not appropriate cuts for the Instant Pot. They are lean, with less fat and cartilage than other cuts, so they may become rubbery or tough in a high-pressure cooking environment.

◼ Seafood

Seafood, ranging from fish like salmon and cod to shellfish such as clams, mussels, and shrimp, are strongly emphasized and encouraged on the Mediterranean diet. Packed with lean protein, seafood is a powerhouse that also provides a variety of nutrients such as omega-3 fatty acids, zinc, and iron. Research shows that omega-3 fatty acids can help reduce inflammation and may help lower the risk of chronic diseases like heart disease, cancer, and arthritis.

Servings: Aim for two or three servings of seafood on a weekly basis. One serving is 3 ounces, which is roughly the size of a deck of playing cards.

Instant Pot Tips: Cooking fish and shellfish in an Instant Pot requires precise timing and attention to detail. However, I love that the cooker can be a great tool to create a flavorful sauce that is then used as the poaching liquid for the seafood.

◼ Poultry

Poultry includes chicken, turkey, and duck, all of which can be found in a variety of cuts. Poultry is an excellent source of protein and provides a range of vitamins and minerals, including B vitamins, selenium, and choline.

Servings: Poultry should be eaten in moderation. One or two servings of poultry can be eaten on a weekly basis. One serving is 3 ounces, which is roughly the size of a deck of playing cards.

Instant Pot Tips: The Instant Pot generally works very well with a variety of poultry. Cuts of poultry that have minimal fat— such as boneless, skinless chicken breast— simply need to be cooked with enough liquid to ensure tender, moist, flavorful results.

◼ Eggs

Eggs are a great way to incorporate healthy animal proteins into your diet. One large egg provides 13 essential vitamins and minerals and 6 grams of high-quality protein. Eggs are particularly beneficial for those who do not eat poultry or meat.

Servings: Eggs should be eaten in moderation. One or two large eggs can be eaten three or four times per week.

Instant Pot Tips: The Instant Pot works very well for specific types of egg cookery, like soft- or hard-boiled, which you will see in this book. Eggs generally won't cook any faster compared to conventional methods, but peeling a hard-boiled egg made in the Instant Pot, versus the stovetop, will convince you it's worthwhile!

Dairy

Dairy foods, including yogurt and cheese, are recommended in moderate amounts in the Mediterranean diet. They are good sources of lean protein and a variety of vitamins and minerals. The dairy group provides essential nutrients like calcium and potassium.

Servings: Aim to consume at least one serving of low-fat dairy daily. One serving equates to 1 cup of plain yogurt or Greek yogurt. Full-fat dairy, like cheese, should be eaten in moderation, or two or three servings on a weekly basis. One serving of cheese equates to 1½ ounces.

Instant Pot Tips: Dairy, like milk or cream, breaks under pressure unless it is part of a batter. As such, any recipes using these ingredients will typically add them at the end after the pressure-cooking time has ended.

Red Meat

Red meat—such as beef, pork, and lamb—can be part of the Mediterranean diet, especially lean, unprocessed cuts of meat. In just 3 ounces, red meat, such as beef, provides 10 essential nutrients, including protein, vitamin B_{12}, zinc, iron, and selenium.

Servings: Keep red meat to one or two servings on a weekly basis. One serving is 3 ounces, which is roughly the size of a deck of playing cards.

Instant Pot Tips: The Instant Pot is an amazing appliance when it comes to tougher cuts of meat that are typically braised and take hours to cook conventionally, such as brisket, chuck roast, veal shanks, or lamb shoulder, to name a few. Using the Instant Pot cuts down on cooking time significantly, seals in flavor, and creates tender, tasty results.

SEAFOOD AND THE INSTANT POT

Pressure cooking seafood can be a great way to get a healthy, delicious meal on the table in minimal time. However, fish and shellfish do require more attention and precise timing to avoid overcooking and becoming tough or rubbery. When preparing seafood, be sure to follow the specific time, pressure, and cooking guidelines in the recipe.

Some shellfish, like mussels or clams, can typically be added to the pressure cooker and steamed or cooked on low for a short time.

Other shellfish, like shrimp, often taste best when added to the pressure cooker after a sauce has been made. They are simply sautéed in the inner pot after the sauce has completed its pressure-cooking time.

Heartier fish, including salmon, tuna, and cod, purchased in fillets or as a whole fish, work beautifully in the Instant Pot.

THE MEDITERRANEAN PANTRY

Getting your Mediterranean pantry together does not require a lot of difficult-to-find or expensive ingredients. Many of these essentials are likely to be in your home already!

Oils

Olive oil is a staple in the Mediterranean diet and the principal source of fat used for cooking, baking, and dressings. It is known for its heart-healthy monounsaturated fat content and anti-inflammatory properties. Olive oil will be your main go-to oil. Regular olive oil typically has a milder flavor and is best for all-purpose cooking. Extra-virgin olive oil can be used for some cooking, but it has a lower smoke point and a more fruity, tangy, or bold flavor that can truly shine as a finishing oil or as part of dressings, dips, or sauces. For a more neutral flavor, canola, avocado, and sunflower oil can be used. Oil should be tightly closed and stored in a cool, dark place.

Nuts and Seeds

Nuts and seeds are good sources of healthy fats, plant-based protein, dietary fiber, and a variety of other nutrients. A study in the *American Journal of Clinical Nutrition* found that people who ate three servings of nuts on a weekly basis had lower indications of inflammation. The Mediterranean diet uses a wide variety of nuts and seeds, but in this book you will most often see almonds, walnuts, pine nuts, and pistachios.

Nuts and seeds are delicious as snacks, but they are also a great addition to many recipes to enhance the flavor, texture, and nutrition of a dish. In general, nuts and seeds are best stored in airtight containers in the refrigerator or freezer due to their high oil content.

Spices and Herbs

Herbs and spices are used to season or add flavor to dishes, which reduces the amount of added salt needed. Herbs used in cooking are typically leaves and stems, and spices are derived from bark, fruit, seeds, or other parts of trees or shrubs. For example, nutmeg is a seed and cinnamon is bark. It is truly amazing what herbs and spices can do. Taken on their own, potatoes may taste fairly bland; but add some tarragon and black pepper, and you have a whole new experience.

You may be familiar with many of the Mediterranean herbs and spices in this book, such as parsley, basil, and mint. However, I have included some that may be new to you.

Za'atar is a spice mixture of dried thyme, sesame seeds, and sumac. You can easily mix your own za'atar spice blend if you like.

Sumac is a dried and ground spice that is typically dark red and has a citrus flavor.

Harissa is a chili paste or red pepper paste that is most often found in ready-made glass jars or tubes. It is often found in the international aisle of your grocery store but is also available online.

INDULGING THE MEDITERRANEAN WAY

The Mediterranean diet is a lifestyle. Moderation and approaching food in a healthy, balanced way are main focal points. It also encourages fostering community and making meals social occasions. As such, savoring meals among family and friends can include enjoying an occasional glass or two of wine or a reasonable portion of dessert. As always, moderation is the key component.

Wine: Making meals a social occasion is part of the Mediterranean lifestyle. One serving is 5 ounces, and having a few glasses per week is reasonable.

Added sugar: Sometimes adding sugar to a dish is essential, as we will see in some of the dessert recipes. Added sugar is about 7 grams per serving. Limit yourself to five servings of added sugar per week.

THE BOOK'S RECIPES

For me, part of the joy of cooking is creating recipes for others to enjoy and being able to experiment and try new things. And guess what? Experimenting in the kitchen can help build your cooking knowledge and confidence, too! This section introduces you to the recipes to come, including the meanings of the labels, tips, and Instant Pot timing instructions.

Labels

To help you identify recipes that cater to specific dietary needs, look for the following labels.

Dairy-Free: Recipes that are free of cow's milk dairy products.

Gluten-Free: Recipes that are free of gluten. Be sure to check the ingredient labels for items like oats to ensure that they are processed in a gluten-free facility.

Cook, Release, and Total Times

The following is a brief explanation of each time-related part of a recipe as it relates to Instant Pot cooking time.

Prep Time: This is the amount of active time spent to prep ingredients, such as chopping, peeling, and slicing.

Pressure Cook: This is the amount of active pressure cooking time.

Pressure Release: Quick release does not add any time, but natural release is indicated here with a specific amount of time.

Total Time: This is the total time to complete the entire recipe and encompasses prep time, sauté time, pressure cook time, simmering time, release time, and an additional 5 or 10 minutes to get to either low or high pressure.

Recipe Tips

The following tips are meant to help navigate the Instant Pot, the Mediterranean diet, and the recipes themselves.

Helpful Hack: Offers tips or tricks to make the prep, cooking process, or recipe easier or more efficient.

Simple Swap: Highlights ingredients that may be swapped out for a variety of reasons, like allergies or to change the flavor profile.

Troubleshooting Tip: Addresses potential Instant Pot issues that may pertain to that recipe.

Save for Later: Suggestions for storing or freezing leftovers.

Let's get Instant Pot pressure cooking!

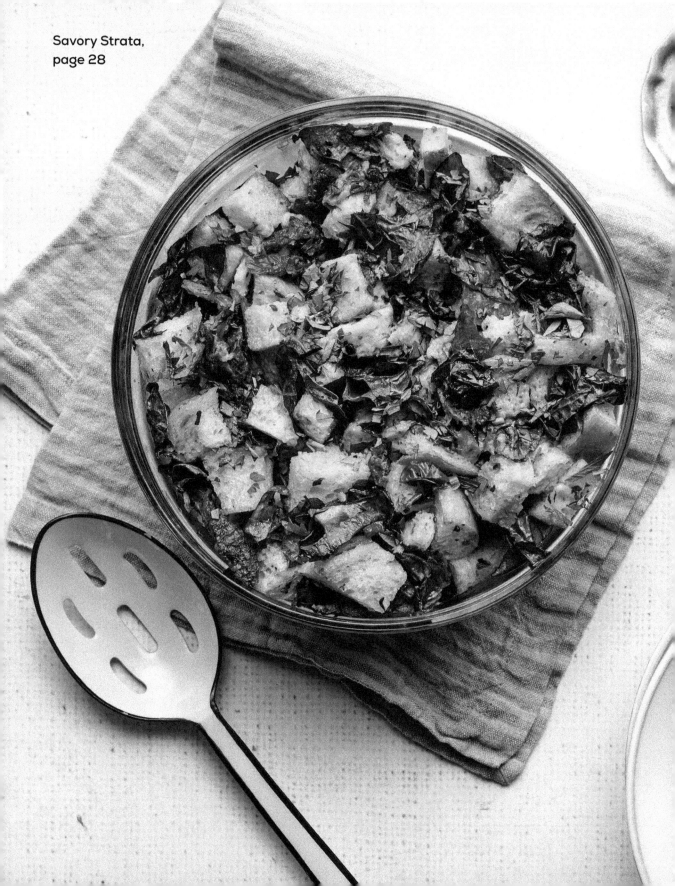

Savory Strata,
page 28

CHAPTER THREE

BREAKFAST

Almond Butter Oatmeal 24

Egg Bites. 25

Yogurt Parfait 26

Savory Strata. 28

Zucchini Frittata 30

Coddled Eggs with Spinach 31

Egg Salad with Avocado. 32

ALMOND BUTTER OATMEAL

**DAIRY-FREE,
GLUTEN-FREE**

Serves 6

Prep time: 5 minutes
Pressure cook:
10 to 13 minutes high
pressure
Pressure release:
10 minutes natural,
then quick
Total time: 35 to
40 minutes

PER SERVING:
Calories: 290; Fat: 13g;
Carbohydrates: 35g; Fiber:
6g; Sugar: 10g; Protein: 10g;
Sodium: 6mg

3¾ cups water
1¼ cups steel-cut oats
½ cup almond butter
**½ cup chopped dried
   apricots**

Oats are a great source of complex carbohydrates, dietary fiber, plant-based protein, and iron—perfect to get you going in the morning. I've paired these oats with almond butter and dried apricots, but feel free to swap them out for your favorite nut or seed butter and dried fruit.

1. In the Instant Pot, combine the water and oats. Stir well. Secure the lid and cook on high pressure for 10 minutes. (For creamier oats, cook on high pressure for 13 minutes.)

2. After cooking, let the pressure release naturally for 10 minutes, then quick release the remaining pressure. Unlock and remove the lid.

3. Stir in the almond butter and apricots (or feel free to swap them out for your favorite nut or seed butter and dried fruit). Serve warm.

SAVE FOR LATER: Let the oats cool for 20 minutes. Cover and refrigerate for up to 1 week. To reheat, scoop out individual servings of the cooked oats. Add 1 tablespoon of water or milk to the chilled oats. Reheat in either a small pot over medium-low heat or in the microwave for about 2 minutes.

EGG BITES

GLUTEN-FREE
Serves 3
Prep time: 10 minutes
Pressure cook:
8 minutes high
pressure
Pressure release:
5 minutes natural,
then quick
Total time: 30 to
35 minutes

PER SERVING: Calories: 180;
Fat: 12g; Carbohydrates: 2g;
Fiber: 0g; Sugar: 2g;
Protein: 15g; Sodium: 380mg

6 large eggs
¼ cup reduced-fat milk
2 asparagus spears,
thinly sliced
⅓ cup crumbled goat
cheese
2 tablespoons
chopped fresh chives
½ teaspoon kosher salt
¼ teaspoon freshly
ground black pepper
1 cup water

With such simple ingredients, these Egg Bites are a cinch to pull together. This recipe features asparagus, goat cheese, and chives. They can be stored in the refrigerator for 3 days and are great on-the-go convenient breakfasts and snacks. I love making Egg Bites on a busy weekday morning, and my family loves having something nourishing on their way out the door.

1. In a medium bowl, beat together the eggs and milk.

2. Stir in the asparagus, goat cheese, chives, salt, and pepper.

3. Ladle or pour the mixture into a 6-bite egg mold and place it on a steam rack.

4. Cover the egg mold tightly with aluminum foil.

5. Pour the water into the Instant Pot, then carefully place the steam rack and egg mold in the pot. Secure the lid and cook on high pressure for 8 minutes.

6. After cooking, let the pressure release naturally for 5 minutes, then quick release the remaining pressure. Unlock and remove the lid.

7. Carefully remove the steam rack and egg mold. Using a spatula or fork, pop the egg bites out of the mold. Serve warm or at room temperature.

SIMPLE SWAP: Egg Bites are a super versatile breakfast option. Feel free to swap out the asparagus, goat cheese, and chives for whatever vegetables, cheese, and herbs you like! You can also make this dairy-free by using plant-based milk and removing the cheese entirely.

YOGURT PARFAIT

GLUTEN-FREE
Serves 2
Prep time: 10 minutes
Total time: 10 minutes

PER SERVING: Calories: 180;
Fat: 8g; Carbohydrates: 19g;
Fiber: 2g; Sugar: 14g;
Protein: 9g; Sodium: 95mg

2 cups Plain Yogurt
   (page 137) or
   store-bought plain
   yogurt
1 cup fresh or frozen
   blueberries
1 teaspoon honey
¼ cup sliced almonds
¼ cup shelled
   pistachios
2 mint sprigs, for
   garnish (optional)

This scrumptious dish calls for plain yogurt that can be made in the Instant Pot. However, plain regular or Greek yogurt purchased at your local grocery store works just as well! Instead of buying a flavored yogurt, buy plain yogurt and add fruit and natural sweeteners like honey. It's a great way to boost flavor and nutrients without all the added sugar. Warming spices like cinnamon, nutmeg, and ginger are also a great addition to this delightful breakfast treat.

1. In a medium bowl, mash together the yogurt, blueberries, and honey.

2. In 2 small serving bowls or clear lowball glasses, layer the yogurt mixture, almonds, and pistachios in any order you like.

3. Garnish with the mint (if using).

SIMPLE SWAP: Use any berries you like or a mixture of several. If using strawberries, be sure to slice or dice them before mashing with the yogurt. Maple syrup is also a great option to sweeten the yogurt a bit in place of the honey; or opt for sugar-free and do not add any sweetener. To transform this into a delectable dessert, add some toasted coconut and chocolate shavings.

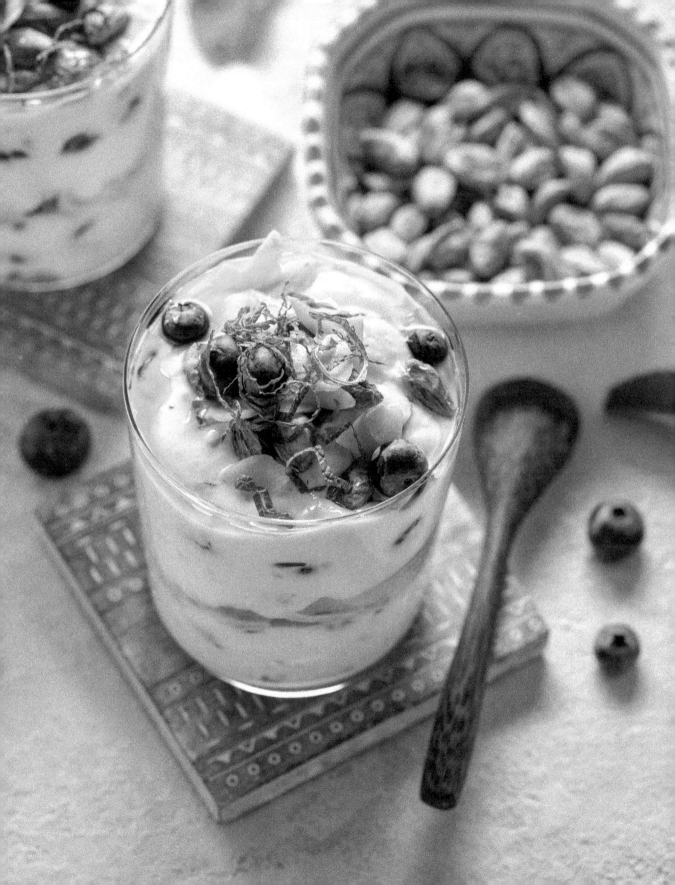

SAVORY STRATA

Serves 6
Prep time: 15 minutes, plus 2 hours to chill
Pressure cook: 25 minutes high pressure
Pressure release: 10 minutes natural, then quick
Total time: 1 hour, plus 2 hours to chill

PER SERVING: Calories: 270; Fat: 6g; Carbohydrates: 40g; Fiber: 2g; Sugar: 2g; Protein: 14g; Sodium: 700mg

This Italian-inspired Savory Strata is easy to throw together before you go to bed. Simply place it in the Instant Pot the next day, and you've got a delicious one-pot dish that's perfect for overnight guests or weekend brunch. It's also a great way to use up some vegetables, cheese, or bread. Looking for something to do with that two- to three-day-old bread? Make a strata!

1 cup Vegetable Stock (page 140) or store-bought vegetable stock
4 large eggs
1½ teaspoons Italian seasoning
½ teaspoon kosher salt
¼ teaspoon freshly ground black pepper
¼ teaspoon red pepper flakes
4 cups cubed sourdough bread
1 bunch Swiss chard, stemmed, leaves chopped
⅓ cup oil-packed sun-dried tomatoes, chopped
⅓ cup grated Parmesan cheese
Olive oil cooking spray, for coating the soufflé dish
1½ cups water
¼ cup chopped fresh parsley, for garnish (optional)

1. In a large bowl, beat together the stock, eggs, Italian seasoning, salt, pepper, and red pepper flakes.

2. Mix in the bread, chard, tomatoes, and cheese. Cover and refrigerate for 2 hours or up to overnight.

3. Lightly spray a 2-quart soufflé dish or 7-cup round glass container with cooking spray.

4. Transfer the egg mixture to the dish, cover tightly with aluminum foil, and place on a steam rack.

5. Pour the water into the Instant Pot, then carefully place the steam rack and dish in the pot. Secure the lid and cook on high pressure for 25 minutes.

6. After cooking, let the pressure release naturally for 10 minutes, then quick release the remaining pressure. Unlock and remove the lid.

7. Carefully remove the steam rack and dish.

8. Garnish with the parsley (if using) and serve.

SIMPLE SWAP: Feel free to swap out the Swiss chard and Parmesan for whatever leafy greens and cheese you like! Spinach or kale would work beautifully and pair nicely with feta, goat cheese, or a variety of hard cheeses like Cheddar or Manchego.

ZUCCHINI FRITTATA

GLUTEN-FREE
Serves 4
Prep time: 10 minutes
Pressure cook:
25 minutes low
pressure
**Pressure
release:** Quick
Total time: 40 minutes

PER SERVING: Calories: 185;
Fat: 12g; Carbohydrates: 2g;
Fiber: 1g; Sugar: 2g;
Protein: 15g; Sodium: 400mg

---

8 large eggs
⅓ cup reduced-fat milk
½ teaspoon dried
   thyme
½ teaspoon kosher salt
¼ teaspoon freshly
   ground black pepper
¼ teaspoon ground
   nutmeg
1 cup grated zucchini
   (1 large)
⅓ cup crumbled feta
   cheese
Olive oil cooking spray,
   for coating the
   soufflé dish
1½ cups water

This frittata is more like an egg casserole when prepared in the Instant Pot, but it is still delicious no matter what you call it. I love the combination of zucchini and feta, and the nutmeg adds a little something special to the mix. Do not swap out the cow's milk for plant-based milk, which is too thin and will produce a different result.

1. In a large bowl, beat together the eggs, milk, thyme, salt, pepper, and nutmeg.

2. Mix in the zucchini and cheese.

3. Lightly spray a 2-quart soufflé dish or 7-cup round glass container with cooking spray.

4. Transfer the egg mixture to the dish, cover tightly with aluminum foil, and place on a steam rack.

5. Pour the water into the Instant Pot, then carefully place the steam rack and dish in the pot. Secure the lid, and cook on low pressure for 25 minutes.

6. After cooking, quick release the pressure. Unlock and remove the lid.

7. Carefully remove the steam rack and serve.

SIMPLE SWAP: Yellow squash or another vegetable you like may be swapped in for the zucchini. However, be sure to grate it so that the cooking time and water content stays the same.

CODDLED EGGS WITH SPINACH

GLUTEN-FREE
Serves 4
Prep time: 10 minutes
Pressure cook:
4 minutes low pressure
Pressure release: Quick
Total time: 20 minutes

PER SERVING: Calories: 100;
Fat: 7g; Carbohydrates: 1g;
Fiber: 0g; Sugar: 0g;
Protein: 9g; Sodium: 315mg

Olive oil cooking spray,
  for coating the
  ramekins
1 cup chopped baby
  spinach
¼ cup grated
  Parmesan cheese
2 teaspoons za'atar
½ teaspoon kosher salt
½ teaspoon freshly
  ground black pepper
4 large eggs
1 cup water

Poached eggs are a much-loved breakfast or brunch favorite, but the Instant Pot is not the appliance to use. Next best thing? Coddled eggs! I love the look and taste of these individual servings of coddled eggs. Serve these eggs with a side of crusty bread to mop up the yolks.

1. Lightly spray 4 ramekins with cooking spray.

2. Divide the spinach, cheese, za'atar, salt, and pepper equally among the ramekins.

3. Crack 1 egg into each ramekin, cover tightly with aluminum foil, and place on a steam rack. (The ramekins may need to be stacked slightly, but be sure not to stack them so that one completely covers another.)

4. Pour the water into the Instant Pot, then carefully place the steam rack and ramekins in the pot. Secure the lid and cook on low pressure for 4 minutes.

5. After cooking, quick release the pressure. Unlock and remove the lid.

6. Carefully remove the steam rack and ramekins. Serve immediately.

SIMPLE SWAP: Coddled eggs taste great with a range of mix-ins. Try chopped Swiss chard with Manchego or grated summer squash with goat cheese. You can also skip the mix-ins altogether and just cook the eggs on their own with some spices and 1 teaspoon of whole milk or cream for some richness.

EGG SALAD WITH AVOCADO

DAIRY-FREE
Serves 4
Prep time: 15 minutes
Total time: 15 minutes

PER SERVING: Calories: 235;
Fat: 11g; Carbohydrates: 24g;
Fiber: 4g; Sugar: 4g;
Protein: 11g; Sodium: 380mg

1 ripe avocado, pitted,
   peeled, and diced
4 Hard-Boiled Eggs
   (page 136), peeled
   and chopped
⅓ cup chopped fresh
   dill
⅓ cup chopped fresh
   parsley
⅓ cup chopped fresh
   chives
Juice of 1 lemon
½ teaspoon kosher salt
¼ teaspoon freshly
   ground black pepper
4 whole-wheat or
   sourdough bread
   slices, toasted

Avocado has long been a staple in the Mediterranean diet. With healthy fats and a ton of fiber, this plant-based treasure is a natural fit. So why add eggs to your avocado toast? Protein! One large egg has 6 grams of protein and a lot of other great nutrients, including choline, vitamin B_{12}, and biotin. Together, they're a perfect combination.

1. In a medium bowl, mash the avocado.

2. Add the eggs, dill, parsley, chives, lemon juice, salt, and pepper. Mix together, keeping a chunky consistency.

3. Serve the egg salad with the toasted bread.

HELPFUL HACK: Use an egg slicer to quickly chop the eggs. Simply place a hard-boiled egg in an egg slicer and slice through. Then turn the egg 90 degrees and slice through the other way.

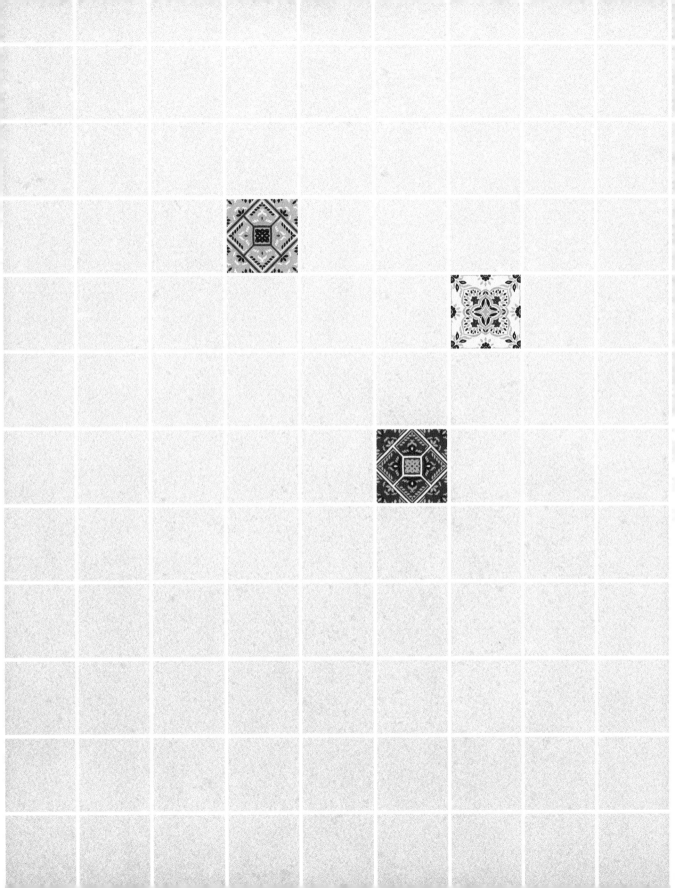

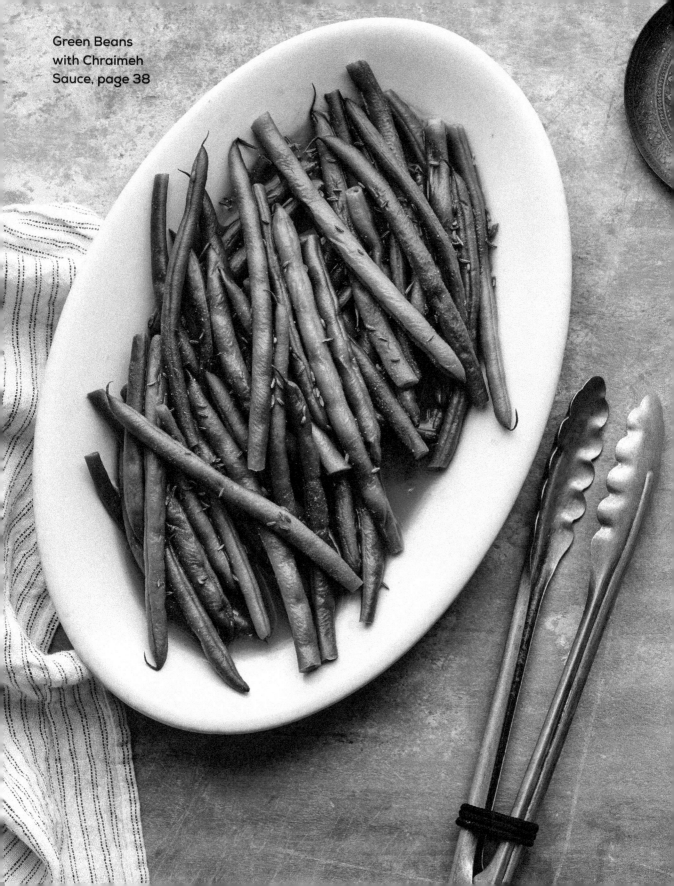

Green Beans
with Chraimeh
Sauce, page 38

CHAPTER FOUR

VEGETABLES AND SIDES

Artichokes with Yogurt Aïoli. 36

Eggplant, Summer Squash, and Tomatoes 37

Green Beans with Chraimeh Sauce. 38

Beets with Tahini Yogurt. 39

Potatoes with Greens 40

Smashed Potatoes. 41

Creamy Polenta with Crème Fraîche 42

Smashed Fava Beans with Toast. 43

Bean Salad 44

Greek-Style Lentils 46

Farro with Herby Yogurt. 48

ARTICHOKES WITH YOGURT AÏOLI

GLUTEN-FREE
Serves 2
Prep time: 5 minutes
Pressure cook:
8 minutes high
pressure
**Pressure
release:** Quick
Total time: 20 to
25 minutes

PER SERVING: Calories: 125;
Fat: 1g; Carbohydrates: 23g;
Fiber: 9g; Sugar: 6g;
Protein: 9g; Sodium: 260mg

FOR THE ARTICHOKES
2 large artichokes
1 cup water

FOR THE AIOLI
½ cup Plain Yogurt
(page 137) or
store-bought plain
yogurt
2 tablespoons
chopped fresh chives
1 teaspoon freshly
squeezed lemon juice
1 teaspoon Dijon
mustard
1 garlic clove, grated
¼ teaspoon kosher salt
⅛ teaspoon freshly
ground black pepper

Artichokes—abundant in Greece, Spain, France, and Italy—may seem intimidating but are easy to prepare in the Instant Pot. Once cooked, the outer leaves can be pulled off and enjoyed by gently using your teeth to scrape off the buttery under-side of the leaves. Beyond the outer leaves, you'll want to remove the purple-topped inner leaves and the fuzzy inner choke that sits on top of the heart. (Eat the artichoke heart—it's the best part!)

TO MAKE THE ARTICHOKES

1. Using kitchen shears, cut off the stem of the arti-chokes, and trim about 1 inch off the tip and the spiky outer leaves.

2. Pour the water into the Instant Pot and place a steam rack inside.

3. Place the artichokes on the steam rack. Secure the lid and cook on high pressure for 8 minutes.

4. After cooking, quick release the pressure. Unlock and remove the lid.

TO MAKE THE AIOLI

5. While the artichokes are cooking, in a small bowl, whisk together the yogurt, chives, lemon juice, mustard, garlic, salt, and pepper. Refrigerate until the artichokes are ready to eat.

6. Serve the artichokes with the aïoli on the side for dipping.

EGGPLANT, SUMMER SQUASH, AND TOMATOES

DAIRY-FREE, GLUTEN-FREE

Serves 4

Prep time: 15 minutes

Pressure cook: 4 minutes high pressure

Pressure release: Quick

Total time: 30 to 35 minutes

1 teaspoon extra-virgin olive oil

1 eggplant, diced (1 pound)

2 summer squash, diced (1 pound)

1 onion, diced

2 garlic cloves, minced

1 (14½-ounce) can low-sodium diced tomatoes

½ cup water, Vegetable Stock (page 140)

2 tablespoons freshly squeezed lemon juice

2 teaspoons dried oregano

2 teaspoons Italian seasoning

¾ teaspoon kosher salt

⅛ teaspoon freshly ground black pepper

1 bay leaf

This recipe is a variation of the French dish ratatouille. Try this recipe with any variety of eggplant or summer squash. Top this dish with toasted nuts or cheese, and serve over Basic Brown Rice (page 134) for a vegetarian meal. If you don't have time to make the Vegetable Stock (page 140), store bought is fine.

1. Press the sauté button on the Instant Pot, allow it to heat up, then pour in the oil.

2. Add the eggplant, squash, and onion. Sauté for about 3 minutes, or until softened.

3. Add the garlic and sauté for 30 seconds, or until fragrant.

4. Add the tomatoes with their juices, water, lemon juice, oregano, Italian seasoning, salt, pepper, and bay leaf. Mix well. Press the cancel button to stop cooking.

5. Secure the lid and cook on high pressure for 4 minutes.

6. After cooking, quick release the pressure. Unlock and remove the lid. Serve warm.

SAVE FOR LATER: This recipe is easily batched up and saved for a future meal. Put the leftovers into containers, and refrigerate for up to 5 days or freeze for up to 3 months.

PER SERVING: Calories: 100; Fat: 2g; Carbohydrates: 19g; Fiber: 6g; Sugar: 12g; Protein: 4g; Sodium: 250mg

GREEN BEANS WITH CHRAIMEH SAUCE

DAIRY-FREE, GLUTEN-FREE

Serves 4
Prep time: 15 minutes
Pressure cook: 1 minute low pressure
Pressure release: Quick
Total time: 20 to 25 minutes

PER SERVING: Calories: 95; Fat: 4g; Carbohydrates: 15g; Fiber: 4g; Sugar: 9g; Protein: 3g; Sodium: 325mg

1 tablespoon avocado oil
5 garlic cloves, sliced
1 tablespoon caraway seeds
1 tablespoon ground cumin
2 teaspoons sweet paprika
1 teaspoon ground cinnamon
3 tablespoons tomato paste
Juice of 1 lime
2 teaspoons honey
1 teaspoon kosher salt
1 cup water
1 pound green beans, trimmed

I first came across chraimeh sauce at a Libyan restaurant many years ago and have been making different versions of it ever since. Though it has roots in North Africa and Libya, variations can be found throughout the Mediterranean region. Traditionally, it is very spicy and often served with fish. My version is more mellow, but if you'd like to kick up the heat, add some cayenne and swap out the sweet paprika for hot or smoked paprika. In addition to green beans, chraimeh sauce is delicious paired with other vegetables, meat, poultry, fish, or some crusty bread.

1. Press the sauté button on the Instant Pot, allow it to heat up, then pour in the oil.

2. Add the garlic, caraway seeds, cumin, paprika, and cinnamon. Sauté for about 1 minute, or until fragrant.

3. Add the tomato paste, lime juice, honey, and salt. Sauté for 30 seconds.

4. Add the water and mix well.

5. Add the green beans and mix together. Press the cancel button to stop cooking.

6. Secure the lid and cook on low pressure for 1 minute.

7. After cooking, quick release the pressure. Unlock and remove the lid.

8. Pour the green beans and sauce into a serving dish and serve immediately or at room temperature.

BEETS WITH TAHINI YOGURT

GLUTEN-FREE
Serves 4
Prep time: 15 minutes
Pressure cook:
20 minutes high
pressure
**Pressure
release:** Quick
Total time: 55 minutes

PER SERVING: Calories: 210;
Fat: 12g; Carbohydrates: 19g;
Fiber: 5g; Sugar: 13g; Protein:
9g; Sodium: 390mg

FOR THE BEETS
1 pound beets,
  trimmed
1 cup water

**FOR THE
TAHINI YOGURT**
½ cup Plain Yogurt
  (page 137) or
  store-bought
  plain yogurt
⅓ cup tahini
2 tablespoons freshly
  squeezed lemon juice
2 tablespoons water
¾ teaspoon kosher salt
½ teaspoon maple
  syrup
¼ teaspoon ground
  cumin
⅛ teaspoon cayenne
  pepper

Beets are delicious, nutritious, and easy to make in the Instant Pot. Wild beets originated in northern Africa and Europe along the Mediterranean Sea. These earthy root vegetables can be found in a range of colors, including purple, pink, golden, white, and red-and-white striped. And be sure to save those beet greens; they'll work beautifully in Savory Strata (page 28). The tahini yogurt can be easily batched up and saved for a future meal.

TO MAKE THE BEETS

1. Fill a bowl with ice water.

2. Pour 1 cup of water into the Instant Pot. Place the beets in a steamer basket or on a steam rack in the pot. Secure the lid and cook on high pressure for 20 minutes.

3. After cooking, quick release the pressure. Unlock and remove the lid.

4. Transfer the beets to the ice water bath, and let cool for 10 minutes.

5. Peel the beets by gently rubbing them with your fingers to remove the peel. Cut into quarters or rounds.

TO MAKE THE TAHINI YOGURT

6. While the beets are cooking, in a small mixing bowl, whisk together the yogurt, tahini, lemon juice, water, salt, maple syrup, cumin, and cayenne. Refrigerate until the beets are ready to eat.

7. Serve the beets topped with the tahini yogurt, or serve with the yogurt on the side for dipping.

POTATOES WITH GREENS

**DAIRY-FREE,
GLUTEN-FREE**

Serves 4

Prep time: 15 minutes

Pressure cook:
7 minutes high
pressure

**Pressure
release:** Quick

Total time: 30 to
35 minutes

PER SERVING: Calories: 180;
Fat: 2g; Carbohydrates: 39g;
Fiber: 7g; Sugar: 6g;
Protein: 9g; Sodium: 320mg

---

1 teaspoon extra-virgin
    olive oil

5 garlic cloves, sliced

2 bunches kale,
    stemmed and
    chopped

1½ pounds small new
    potatoes, halved

1 cup water, Vegetable
    Stock (page 140),
    or store-bought
    vegetable stock

2 tablespoons freshly
    squeezed lemon juice

1 teaspoon kosher salt

¼ teaspoon freshly
    ground black pepper

There are many different varieties of potatoes, but
I find that small, waxy types work best in this dish.
This is because they are less starchy and retain
their shape and structure better in the Instant Pot.
Look for mini or small potatoes that are one bite
when cut in half. Waxy potato varieties include
new potatoes, red bliss, fingerlings, and blue or
red potatoes, to name a few. Other hearty greens,
such as collard greens or mustard greens, can be
used in place of the kale if preferred.

1. Press the sauté button on the Instant Pot, allow it
   to heat up, then pour in the oil.

2. Add the garlic and sauté for about 30 seconds, or
   until fragrant.

3. Add the kale, potatoes, water, lemon juice, salt,
   and pepper. Mix well. Press the cancel button to
   stop cooking.

4. Secure the lid and cook on high pressure for
   7 minutes.

5. After cooking, quick release the pressure. Unlock
   and remove the lid. Serve warm.

HELPFUL HACK: Pre-chopped kale can be used to cut
down on prep time.

SMASHED POTATOES

**DAIRY-FREE,
GLUTEN-FREE**

Serves 4
Prep time: 5 minutes
Pressure cook:
15 minutes high
pressure
**Pressure
release:** Quick
Total time: 55 minutes

PER SERVING: Calories: 175;
Fat: 7g; Carbohydrates: 29g;
Fiber: 3g; Sugar: 3g;
Protein: 5g; Sodium: 280mg

1 cup water
1½ pounds mini
   potatoes
2 tablespoons
   extra-virgin olive oil
1 teaspoon kosher salt
¼ teaspoon freshly
   ground black pepper
6 rosemary sprigs

Is there anything better than potatoes that are crispy on the outside and tender on the inside? This recipe is a delight and a crowd-pleaser for sure. Don't let the double cooking methods deter you; it's well worth it and still a cinch to prepare! Pair with Lamb Meat Loaf with Tahini Sauce (page 108) and a fresh salad for a delicious, well-balanced meal.

1. Pour the water into the Instant Pot. Place the potatoes in a steamer basket in the pot. Secure the lid and cook on high pressure for 15 minutes.

2. Preheat the oven to 450°F. Line a baking sheet with aluminum foil or parchment paper.

3. After cooking, quick release the pressure. Unlock and remove the lid.

4. Put the potatoes on the prepared baking sheet, and toss with the oil, salt, and pepper.

5. Spread the potatoes out on the baking sheet in a single layer, then using the bottom of a glass or measuring cup, flatten or smash them.

6. Place the rosemary sprigs on the baking sheet.

7. Transfer the baking sheet to the oven and roast for 25 minutes, or until the potatoes are golden brown. Remove from the oven. Serve immediately.

SIMPLE SWAP: Change up the herbs and spices here however you like. Toss the potatoes with cayenne, garlic powder, and onion powder in place of the salt and pepper, or use crushed garlic cloves instead of–or in addition to–the rosemary.

CREAMY POLENTA WITH CRÈME FRAÎCHE

GLUTEN-FREE
Serves 6
Prep time: 10 minutes
Pressure cook:
8 minutes high
pressure
Pressure release:
20 minutes natural,
then quick
Total time: 55 minutes

PER SERVING:
Calories: 225; Fat: 15g;
Carbohydrates: 20g;
Fiber: 3g; Sugar: 1g;
Protein: 6g; Sodium: 320mg

4 cups Vegetable
  Stock (page 140)
  or store-bought
  vegetable stock
3 tablespoons
  unsalted butter,
  cubed
½ teaspoon kosher salt
1 cup coarse-ground
  yellow polenta or
  corn grits
½ cup grated Pecorino
  Romano cheese
⅓ cup crème fraîche
¼ teaspoon freshly
  ground black pepper

Polenta is a classic Italian side dish that is made from cooked cornmeal or corn grits. A widespread belief is that polenta takes a lot of time and whisking to be cooked properly, but the Instant Pot makes it easy. Serve it as a side dish, or use it in place of pasta. Eggplant, Summer Squash, and Tomatoes (page 37) would be a perfect topper!

1. In the Instant Pot, combine the stock, butter, and salt. Press the sauté button. Melt the butter, and simmer for about 5 minutes.

2. Stir in the polenta and whisk constantly for 2 minutes. Press the cancel button to stop cooking.

3. Secure the lid and cook on high pressure for 8 minutes.

4. After cooking, let the pressure release naturally for 20 minutes, then quick release the remaining pressure. Unlock and remove the lid.

5. Stir in the cheese, crème fraîche, and pepper. Continue to stir together for about 1 minute, or until the cheese has melted and the polenta smooths out a bit. Transfer to a serving dish.

SIMPLE SWAP: Can't find crème fraîche? Mascarpone cheese, cream cheese, or sour cream can be used instead.

SMASHED FAVA BEANS WITH TOAST

Serves 6
Prep time: 1 hour, plus overnight to soak
Pressure cook: 7 minutes low pressure
Pressure release: 15 minutes natural, then quick
Total time: 1 hour 30 minutes, plus overnight to soak

PER SERVING: Calories: 370; Fat: 14g; Carbohydrates: 50g; Fiber: 9g; Sugar: 6g; Protein: 16g; Sodium: 620mg

---

1 pound dried fava beans

8 cups water

½ cup minced fresh mint leaves

3 tablespoons extra-virgin olive oil

Grated zest of 1 lemon

Juice of 1 lemon

½ teaspoon kosher salt

½ teaspoon red pepper flakes

½ cup grated Parmesan cheese

12 whole-wheat or sourdough bread slices, toasted

Fava beans, also known as broad beans, are native to North Africa and the Mediterranean region and are used in a variety of recipes. They take some time and care to prepare since they must be soaked and peeled but are well worth it. If you see fresh fava beans at your local farmers' market, they can be swapped in and used in this recipe. If using fresh fava beans, you do not need to soak them overnight.

---

1. Put the fava beans in the Instant Pot, fill with water, then refrigerate overnight or for up to 24 hours.

2. Drain and rinse the beans. Peel the outer skin off each bean.

3. In the Instant Pot, combine the beans and the water. Secure the lid and cook on low pressure for 7 minutes.

4. While the beans are cooking, in a large bowl, mix together the mint, oil, lemon zest, lemon juice, salt, and red pepper flakes.

5. After cooking, let the pressure release naturally for 15 minutes, then quick release the remaining pressure. Unlock and remove the lid. Drain the beans.

6. Add the beans and cheese to the mint mixture. Mix well and smash to your desired consistency.

7. Serve the smashed beans with the toasted bread.

SIMPLE SWAP: Don't want to spend the extra time soaking and peeling or can't find fava beans? Use dried soybeans or frozen shelled edamame instead.

BEAN SALAD

**DAIRY-FREE,
GLUTEN-FREE**

Serves 4
Prep time: 20 minutes
Total time: 20 minutes

PER SERVING:
Calories: 340; Fat: 20g;
Carbohydrates: 32g;
Fiber: 9g; Sugar: 9g;
Protein: 10g; Sodium: 335mg

2 cups Chickpeas
   (page 135) or canned
   chickpeas
½ cup Tahini Dressing
   (page 144)
1 pint cherry tomatoes,
   halved
2 carrots, shaved
1 hothouse cucumber,
   diced
1 red bell pepper, diced
2 celery stalks, diced

A simple salad with a variety of fresh vegetables, beans, and a delicious dressing is a fantastic light lunch or part of a larger meal. The vegetables provide a range of vitamins and minerals, the beans are an excellent source of plant-based protein, and the tahini dressing is chock-full of healthy fats. To add even more protein, fiber, and tasty crunch, garnish this salad with some toasted walnuts or almonds, and top with some fresh chopped parsley.

1. In a large bowl, combine the chickpeas and tahini dressing. Mix well.

2. Add the tomatoes, carrots, cucumber, bell pepper, and celery. Toss together well and serve.

SIMPLE SWAP: Although this recipe calls for cooked chickpeas, also known as garbanzo beans, any beans you like can be used. A variety of vegetables (try green beans, broccoli, or asparagus) would also work well in this fresh salad.

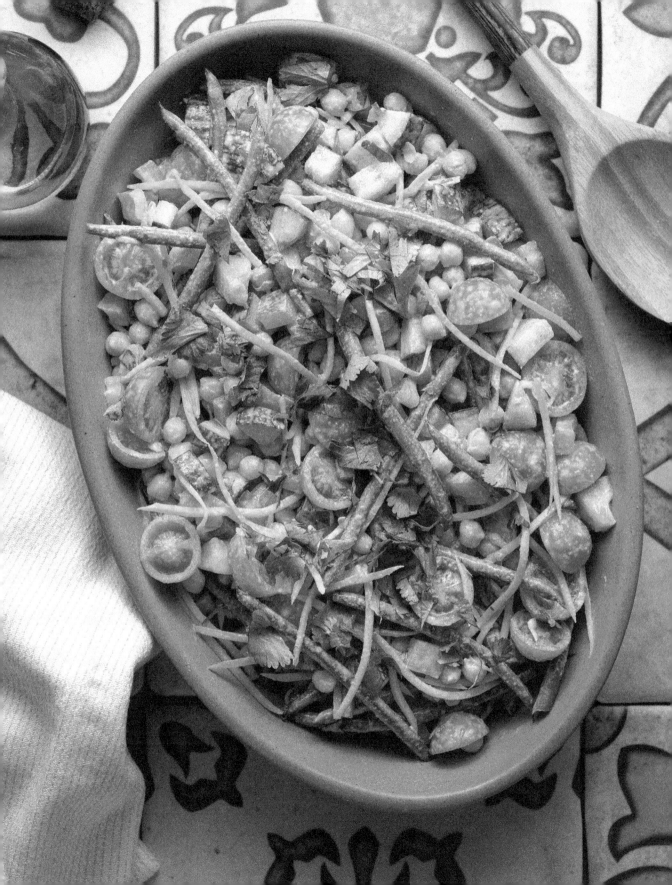

GREEK-STYLE LENTILS

**DAIRY-FREE,
GLUTEN-FREE**

Serves 6
Prep time: 15 minutes
Pressure cook:
20 minutes high
pressure
Pressure release:
10 minutes natural,
then quick
Total time: 1 hour
5 minutes

PER SERVING: Calories: 235;
Fat: 3g; Carbohydrates: 38g;
Fiber: 17g; Sugar: 6g;
Protein: 14g; Sodium: 287mg

Lentils are an excellent source of plant-based protein and iron, making them a perfect alternative to meat. They are a rich source of many vitamins and minerals, including B vitamins, magnesium, zinc, and potassium, as well as dietary fiber. There are dozens of lentil varieties, ranging from black to yellow, red, and green. For this recipe, I prefer green, or French, lentils because they hold their shape well and do not turn mushy in the Instant Pot.

---

1 tablespoon extra-virgin olive oil
1 onion, finely diced
2 carrots, finely diced
2 celery stalks, finely diced
1 teaspoon kosher salt
2 garlic cloves, minced
1 tablespoon tomato paste
1 teaspoon dried oregano
½ teaspoon ground cinnamon
⅛ teaspoon red pepper flakes
2½ cups Vegetable Stock (page 140) or
  store-bought vegetable stock
1½ cups dried French green lentils, picked through
  and rinsed
1 (14½-ounce) can low-sodium diced tomatoes

1. Press the sauté button on the Instant Pot, allow it to heat up, then pour in the oil.

2. Add the onion, carrots, celery, and salt. Sauté, stirring frequently, for 5 minutes, or until softened.

3. Add the garlic and sauté for 30 seconds, or until fragrant.

4. Add the tomato paste, oregano, cinnamon, and red pepper flakes. Sauté for 30 seconds.

5. Add the stock, lentils, and tomatoes with their juices. Mix together. Press the cancel button to stop cooking.

6. Secure the lid and cook on high pressure for 20 minutes.

7. After cooking, let the pressure release naturally for 10 minutes, then quick release the remaining pressure. Unlock and remove the lid.

8. Stir the lentil mixture well and serve.

SIMPLE SWAP: If you have fresh tomatoes, you can chop about 2 cups and use them in place of the canned tomatoes. If you use raw tomatoes, sauté them in step 2 and add an extra ½ cup of stock in step 5.

FARRO WITH HERBY YOGURT

Serves 4
Prep time: 5 minutes
Pressure cook:
25 minutes high
pressure
Pressure release:
10 minutes natural,
then quick
Total time: 50 minutes

PER SERVING: Calories: 215;
Fat: 1g; Carbohydrates: 39g;
Fiber: 4g; Sugar: 4g;
Protein: 10g; Sodium: 390mg

FOR THE FARRO
3 cups water
1 cup farro

**FOR THE
HERBY YOGURT**

1 cup fresh mint leaves
1 cup fresh parsley
⅓ cup buttermilk
Grated zest of 1 lemon
2 tablespoons freshly
    squeezed lemon juice
1 teaspoon kosher salt
¼ teaspoon freshly
    ground black pepper
⅔ cup Plain Yogurt
    (page 137) or
    store-bought plain
    yogurt

Farro is a popular grain throughout Italy. It is a distant cousin of wheat but looks like a jumbo-size grain of brown rice with a flat, cleaved belly and a rounded back. It has a rich, earthy, nutty flavor that pairs beautifully with this herby yogurt. Farro is an excellent source of fiber, plant-based protein, complex carbohydrates, and a range of vitamins and minerals. Pair this dish with a side salad or some roasted vegetables for a delicious vegetarian meal.

TO MAKE THE FARRO

1. In the Instant Pot, combine the water and farro. Secure the lid and cook on high pressure for 25 minutes.

2. After cooking, let the pressure release naturally for 10 minutes, then quick release the remaining pressure. Unlock and remove the lid. Drain the farro.

TO MAKE THE HERBY YOGURT

3. While the farro is cooking, in a blender, combine the mint, parsley, buttermilk, lemon zest, lemon juice, salt, and pepper. Puree, then pour into a bowl.

4. Add the yogurt and whisk together. Refrigerate until the farro is cooked.

5. Add the farro to the yogurt mixture and stir together well. Serve immediately warm, at room temperature, or cold.

SAVE FOR LATER: If you want to save some plain farro to use later, allow it to cool, then transfer to an airtight container and refrigerate for up to 1 week, or freeze for up to 3 months.

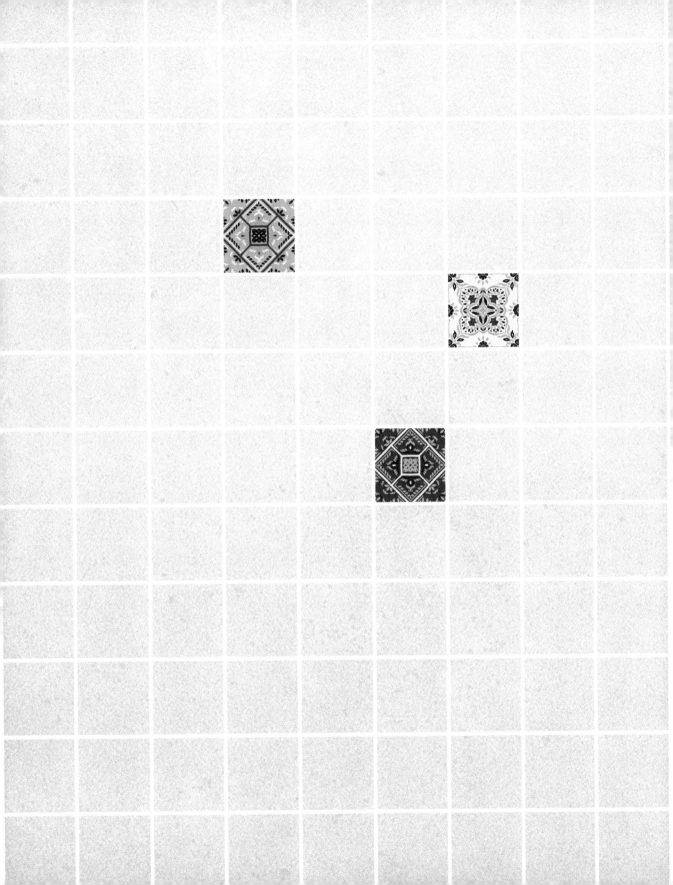

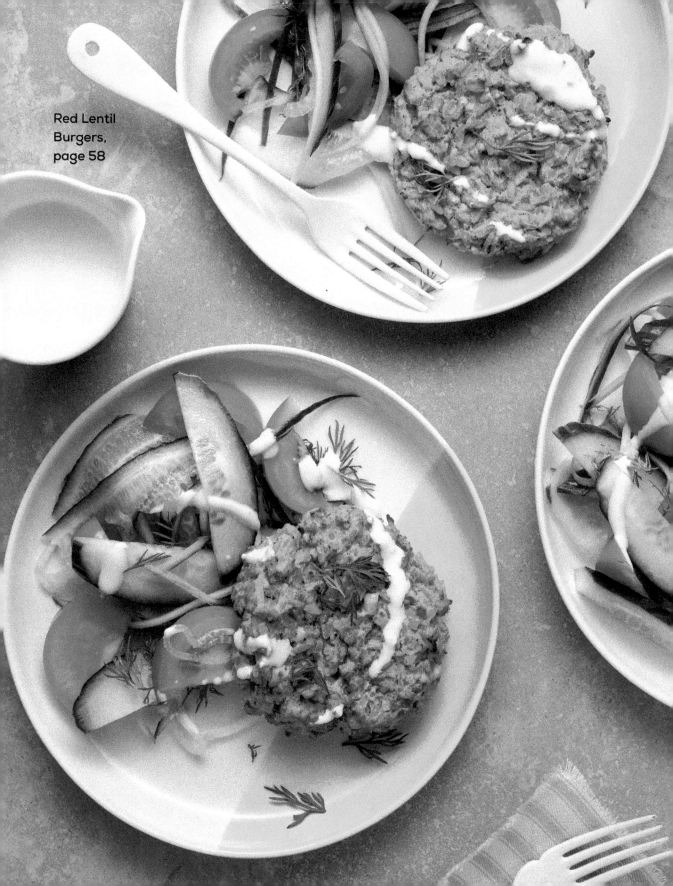

Red Lentil
Burgers,
page 58

CHAPTER FIVE

MEATLESS MAINS

Bean Soup. 52

Lentil and Eggplant Stew 53

Mujadara. 54

Vegetable Bourguignon 56

Red Lentil Burgers. 58

Moroccan Tagine with Butternut Squash and Chickpeas . . . 61

Spiced Chickpea Bowls 63

Risotto with Mushrooms and Asparagus 64

Stuffed Sweet Potatoes 66

Spaghetti Squash with Cherry Tomatoes, Basil, and Feta . . 67

Pasta with Marinara Sauce 68

Jammy Eggs with Hummus and Rice Salad. 69

Lentil Ragù 70

Couscous with Eggplant 72

BEAN SOUP

**DAIRY-FREE,
GLUTEN-FREE**

Serves 10
Prep time: 15 minutes
Pressure cook:
45 minutes high
pressure
Pressure release:
20 minutes natural,
then quick
Total time: 1 hour
40 minutes

1 teaspoon extra-virgin
    olive oil
1 onion, diced
2 celery stalks, diced
2 carrots, diced
4 cups water
4 cups Vegetable
    Stock (page 140)
    or store-bought
    vegetable stock
1 pound dried kidney
    beans
1 tablespoon dried
    oregano
1 teaspoon dried
    thyme
2 bay leaves
1 (14½-ounce) can
    diced tomatoes
3 tablespoons freshly
    squeezed lemon juice
1 teaspoon kosher salt
¼ teaspoon freshly
    ground black pepper

Beans are one of the most common foods eaten worldwide, thanks to their affordability and versatility. My recipe uses kidney beans, but any beans you like will work well and taste great; you can also try a mix of different types of beans or use a "bean soup mix." Beans are an excellent source of plant-based protein, dietary fiber, folate, iron, and magnesium.

1. Press the sauté button on the Instant Pot, allow it to heat up for 1 minute, then pour in the oil.

2. Add the onion, celery, and carrots. Sauté, stirring frequently, for 5 minutes, or until softened.

3. Add the water, stock, beans, parsley, oregano, thyme, and bay leaves. Press the cancel button to stop cooking.

4. Secure the lid and cook on high pressure for 45 minutes.

5. After cooking, let the pressure release naturally for 20 minutes, then quick release the remaining pressure. Unlock and remove the lid.

6. Mix in the tomatoes with their juices, lemon juice, salt, and pepper.

7. Mash some of the beans to thicken, if desired, and serve warm.

SAVE FOR LATER: Portion out the soup into containers, label each container with the name and date, then freeze for up to 6 months.

PER SERVING: Calories: 185; Fat: 1g; Carbohydrates: 33g; Fiber: 13g; Sugar: 4g; Protein: 11g; Sodium: 200mg

LENTIL AND EGGPLANT STEW

GLUTEN-FREE
Serves 4
Prep time: 15 minutes
Pressure cook:
15 minutes high
pressure
Pressure release:
15 minutes natural,
then quick
Total time: 1 hour
5 minutes

PER SERVING: Calories: 320;
Fat: 8g; Carbohydrates: 45g;
Fiber: 20g; Sugar: 9g;
Protein: 15g; Sodium: 300mg

1 red onion, diced
2 tablespoons
  extra-virgin olive oil
1 teaspoon kosher salt
2 tablespoons fresh
  thyme leaves
4 garlic cloves, sliced
¼ teaspoon freshly
  ground black pepper
1 eggplant, diced
  (1½ pounds)
1 pint cherry tomatoes
½ cup white wine
2 cups water
1 cup dried French
  green lentils
Juice of ½ lemon
Crème fraîche, for
  serving (optional)

Eggplant belongs to the nightshade family, along with tomatoes and potatoes. The most popular variety of eggplant looks like a large, pear-shaped egg—get it, "eggplant"—and has a glossy, deep-purple skin and a cream-colored flesh with a spongy consistency when raw. There are several varieties of eggplant available, all of which taste great in this dish.

1. Press the sauté button on the Instant Pot, allow it to heat up, then pour in the onion, oil, and salt. Sauté for 3 minutes, or until the onion has softened.

2. Add the thyme, garlic, and pepper. Sauté for 30 seconds, or until fragrant.

3. Add the eggplant and tomatoes. Sauté for 3 minutes, or until softened.

4. Add the wine and deglaze: Mix well, scrape up any brown bits, and reduce the wine for about 1 minute.

5. Add the water and lentils. Mix well. Press the cancel button to stop cooking.

6. Secure the lid and cook on high pressure for 15 minutes.

7. After cooking, let the pressure release naturally for 15 minutes, then quick release the remaining pressure. Unlock and remove the lid.

8. Add the lemon juice and mix well. If desired, press the sauté button and cook, stirring occasionally, to thicken to the desired consistency.

9. Serve the stew garnished with a dollop of crème fraîche (if using).

MUJADARA

GLUTEN-FREE
Serves 4
Prep time: 15 minutes
Pressure cook:
16 minutes high
pressure
Pressure release:
16 minutes natural,
then quick
Total time: 55 minutes
to 1 hour

PER SERVING:
Calories: 530; Fat: 16g;
Carbohydrates: 77g;
Fiber: 18g; Sugar: 10g;
Protein: 20g; Sodium: 435mg

Mujadara is a popular plant-based protein-rich Middle Eastern dish known throughout Israel, Lebanon, and Egypt, to name a few. It is a variation of rice pilaf made with brown rice, lentils, and caramelized or crispy onions. I've paired this version with yogurt, but feel free to swap it out and top with a fried egg or roasted fish instead.

FOR THE RICE AND LENTILS
1 tablespoon extra-virgin olive oil
4 garlic cloves, smashed and peeled
2 teaspoons ground cumin
1 teaspoon ground coriander
3 cups Vegetable Stock (page 140) or
    store-bought vegetable stock
1 cup long-grain brown rice
1 cup dried French green lentils
1 teaspoon kosher salt
¼ teaspoon freshly ground black pepper
1 bay leaf

FOR THE MUJADARA
⅓ cup vegetable oil or canola oil
2 onions, julienned
½ cup chopped fresh parsley, divided
1 cup Plain Yogurt (page 137) or store-bought
    plain yogurt
Hot sauce, for serving (optional)
Tahini, for serving (optional)

TO MAKE THE RICE AND LENTILS

1. Press the sauté button on the Instant Pot, allow it to heat up, then pour in the oil.

2. Add the garlic, cumin, and coriander. Sauté for 30 seconds, or until fragrant.

3. Add the stock, rice, lentils, salt, pepper, and bay leaf. Mix well. Press the cancel button to stop cooking.

4. Secure the lid and cook on high pressure for 16 minutes.

5. After cooking, let the pressure release naturally for 16 minutes, then quick release the remaining pressure. Unlock and remove the lid.

6. Mix together the rice and lentils, remove the bay leaf, then place the lid askew over the pot to partially cover.

TO MAKE THE MUJADARA

7. While the rice and lentils are cooking, in a large skillet, heat the oil over medium heat. Line a plate with paper towels.

8. Add the onions and cook, stirring occasionally, for 30 minutes, or until golden and cooked to your desired crispness. Remove from the heat and transfer to the prepared plate.

9. Mix half of the onions and ¼ cup of parsley in with the rice and lentils. Transfer to a large serving dish.

10. Serve the mujadara with the remaining onions, ¼ cup of parsley, the yogurt, hot sauce (if using), and tahini (if using) on the side.

TROUBLESHOOTING TIP: The pressure cooking and release timing for this dish is based on long-grain brown rice. If you use a different variety, like short-grain brown rice, the cooking time may change.

VEGETABLE BOURGUIGNON

Serves 4
Prep time: 20 minutes
Pressure cook:
5 minutes high
pressure
**Pressure
release:** Quick
Total time: 1 hour
10 minutes

PER SERVING: Calories: 270;
Fat: 10g; Carbohydrates: 27g;
Fiber: 5g; Sugar: 11g;
Protein: 7g; Sodium: 590mg

Meaty mushrooms are the highlight of this vegetarian spin on the classic French beef stew. Feel free to swap out the carrots and celery for parsnips, turnips, or rutabaga. If you're not concerned about keeping this vegetarian, beef stock is a great substitute for the vegetable stock. Serve this on its own or over Creamy Polenta with Crème Fraîche (page 42).

2 tablespoons extra-virgin olive oil
1 tablespoon unsalted butter
1½ pounds mixed mushrooms, such as cremini, white button, shiitake, sliced
2 celery stalks, diced
2 carrots, diced
1 leek, white and light green parts only, sliced
3 garlic cloves, minced
1 bay leaf
1 teaspoon dried thyme
1 teaspoon kosher salt
¼ teaspoon freshly ground black pepper
1 tablespoon tomato paste
1 tablespoon all-purpose flour
1½ cups red wine
1 (14-ounce bag) frozen pearl onions
1½ cups Vegetable Stock (page 140) or store-bought vegetable stock
1½ tablespoons soy sauce
½ cup chopped fresh parsley, for garnish

1. Press the sauté button on the Instant Pot, allow it to heat up, then pour in the oil and butter.

2. Once the butter has melted, add the mushrooms, celery, carrots, and leek. Sauté, stirring occasionally, for about 15 minutes, or until the mushrooms release most of their moisture.

3. Add the garlic, bay leaf, thyme, salt, and pepper. Cook for 5 minutes, or until fragrant. Try to boil off some of the water from cooking the mushrooms.

4. Add the tomato paste and sauté for 1 minute.

5. Sprinkle the flour over the vegetables.

6. Add the wine and deglaze: Mix well and scrape up any brown bits on the bottom of the pot. Reduce the wine by half, about 5 minutes.

7. Add the onions, stock, and soy sauce. Mix well. Press the cancel button to stop cooking.

8. Secure the lid and cook on high pressure for 5 minutes.

9. After cooking, quick release the pressure. Unlock and remove the lid, then mix well.

10. Press the sauté button and cook, stirring occasionally, until the desired consistency is reached. Press the cancel button to stop cooking.

11. Serve the stew garnished with the parsley.

SIMPLE SWAP: To make this dish gluten-free, swap out the all-purpose flour for gluten-free flour, and use gluten-free tamari in place of the soy sauce.

RED LENTIL BURGERS

**DAIRY-FREE,
GLUTEN-FREE**

Serves 6
Prep time: 20 minutes
Pressure cook:
3 minutes high
pressure
Pressure release:
10 minutes natural,
then quick
Total time: 1 hour
20 minutes

PER SERVING: Calories: 280;
Fat: 8g; Carbohydrates: 41g;
Fiber: 7g; Sugar: 3g;
Protein: 13g; Sodium: 200mg

These plant-based burgers are beautifully golden with fragrant spices. Serve them on their own or topped with Plain Yogurt (page 137), spicy mango chutney, or a refreshing tomato-cucumber salad. I am partial to cashews for this recipe, but any nuts you like will be delicious.

1 tablespoon extra-virgin olive oil
1 onion, finely diced
1 red bell pepper, finely diced
1 tablespoon grated fresh ginger
1 tablespoon ground cumin
2 garlic cloves, minced
1 teaspoon ground coriander
1 teaspoon ground turmeric
1 teaspoon kosher salt
½ teaspoon ground cinnamon
¼ teaspoon freshly ground black pepper
1½ cups water
1 cup dried red lentils
2 cups Basic Brown Rice (page 134)
½ cup chopped toasted cashews
⅓ cup minced fresh cilantro
Juice of ½ lemon

1. Press the sauté button on the Instant Pot, allow it to heat up, then pour in the oil.

2. Add the onion and bell pepper. Sauté for about 3 minutes, or until soft.

3. Add the ginger, cumin, garlic, coriander, turmeric, salt, cinnamon, and pepper. Sauté for 1 minute, or until fragrant.

4. Add the water and lentils. Mix well. Press the cancel button to stop cooking.

5. Secure the lid and cook on high pressure for 3 minutes.

6. After cooking, let the pressure release naturally for 10 minutes, then quick release the remaining pressure. Unlock and remove the lid, then mix well.

7. Preheat the oven to 400°F. Line a baking sheet with parchment paper.

8. Carefully remove the inner pot and put it on a trivet on the counter near the baking sheet.

9. Add the rice, cashews, cilantro, and lemon juice to the lentil mixture. Mix well. Spoon heaping ½-cup portions onto the prepared baking sheet. Using the bottom of the measuring cup or a glass, flatten them out slightly.

10. Transfer the baking sheet to the oven and bake for 30 minutes, or until the patties are slightly golden brown. Remove from the oven. Serve immediately.

SAVE FOR LATER: Put the leftover patties in resealable freezer bags, separated by pieces of parchment or wax paper. Be sure to label the bag with the name of the food and date. These patties should last up to 3 months in the freezer.

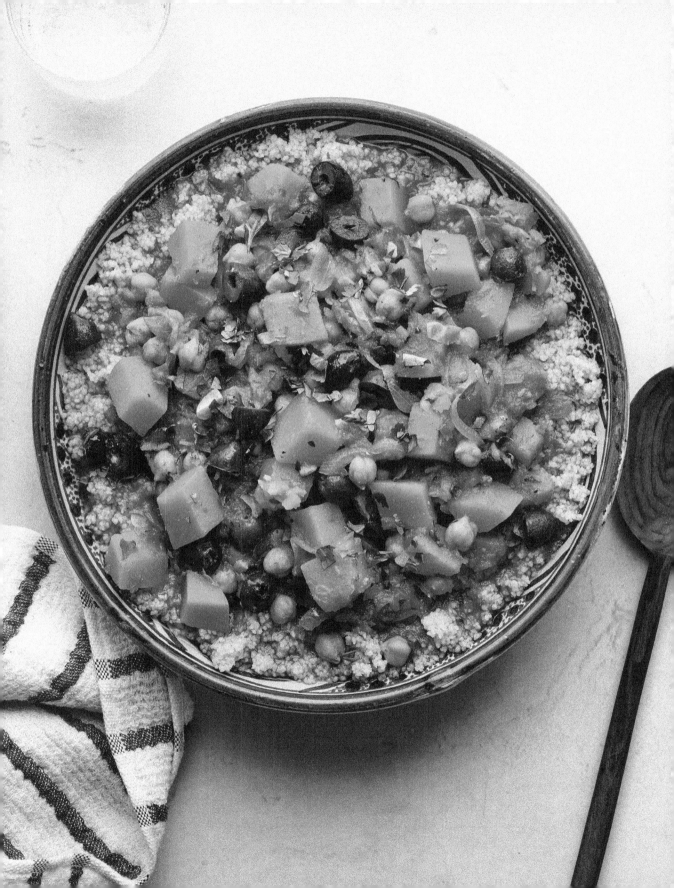

MOROCCAN TAGINE WITH BUTTERNUT SQUASH AND CHICKPEAS

DAIRY-FREE, GLUTEN-FREE

Serves 6

Prep time: 20 minutes, plus 8 hours to soak

Pressure cook: 25 minutes high pressure

Pressure release: Quick

Total time: 1 hour 5 minutes, plus 8 hours to soak

PER SERVING: Calories: 300; Fat: 7g; Carbohydrates: 51g; Fiber: 13g; Sugar: 12g; Protein: 12g; Sodium: 391mg

---

Tagine is a stew-like dish that often contains meat, poultry, or fish and a variety of vegetables or fruit. My version is vegan and full of the plant-based protein powerhouse, chickpeas; a variety of vegetables; and aromatic Moroccan spices. If you like the idea of fruit in your tagine, add ½ cup of raisins or dried apricots in step 6. Serve over some Basic Brown Rice (page 134) or another grain, like couscous, to soak up the delicious liquid.

---

1 tablespoon extra-virgin olive oil

1 onion, julienned

5 garlic cloves, minced

3 (2-inch) strips lemon zest

1 teaspoon ground cumin

¾ teaspoon kosher salt

½ teaspoon ground cinnamon

½ teaspoon ground coriander

⅛ teaspoon cayenne pepper

1 (1½-pound) butternut squash, peeled, seeded, and cut into 1-inch pieces

1 (14½-ounce) can low-sodium diced tomatoes

2 cups Vegetable Stock (page 140) or store-bought vegetable stock

1½ cups dried chickpeas, soaked for 8 hours or overnight

½ cup chopped pitted Kalamata olives

½ cup chopped fresh cilantro

Juice of ½ lemon

continued ➤

1. Press the sauté button on the Instant Pot, allow it to heat up, then pour in the oil.

2. Add the onion and sauté for about 2 minutes, or until softened.

3. Add the garlic and sauté for 30 seconds, or until fragrant.

4. Add the lemon zest, cumin, salt, cinnamon, coriander, and cayenne. Sauté for 30 seconds, or until fragrant.

5. Add the squash and tomatoes with their juices. Mix well and scrape up any brown bits on the bottom of the pot.

6. Add the stock and chickpeas. Mix well. Press the cancel button to stop cooking.

7. Secure the lid and cook on high pressure for 25 minutes.

8. After cooking, quick release the pressure. Unlock and remove the lid, then mix well.

9. Press the sauté button and cook for 5 minutes, reducing the liquid slightly.

10. Add the olives, cilantro, and lemon juice. Mix well. Press the cancel button to stop cooking. Serve immediately.

HELPFUL HACK: Shave off some prep time by purchasing butternut squash already peeled, seeded, and cut into pieces.

SPICED CHICKPEA BOWLS

GLUTEN-FREE
Serves 4
Prep time: 15 minutes
Total time: 15 minutes

PER SERVING: Calories: 330;
Fat: 9g; Carbohydrates: 49g;
Fiber: 14g; Sugar: 14g;
Protein: 16g; Sodium: 250mg

FOR THE YOGURT

1 cup Plain Yogurt
　(page 137) or
　store-bought plain
　yogurt
2 tablespoons freshly
　squeezed lemon juice
½ teaspoon kosher salt
½ teaspoon ground
　cumin
¼ teaspoon ground
　coriander

FOR THE BOWLS

3 cups Chickpeas
　(page 135) or canned
　chickpeas
2 carrots, grated
1 fennel bulb, sliced
1 ripe avocado, pitted,
　peeled, and sliced
¼ cup chopped fresh
　cilantro, for garnish
¼ cup chopped fresh
　parsley, for garnish

These Spiced Chickpea Bowls make for an easy, delicious lunch or light dinner.

TO MAKE THE YOGURT

1. In a small bowl, mix together the yogurt, lemon juice, salt, cumin, and coriander.

TO MAKE THE BOWLS

2. Divide the yogurt mixture among four serving bowls.

3. Divide the chickpeas, carrots, and fennel among the bowls over top of the yogurt.

4. Divide the avocado on top of each serving bowl.

5. Serve the bowls garnished with the cilantro and parsley.

SIMPLE SWAP: If you don't have cooked chickpeas, the canned variety can be used. The chickpeas can also be swapped out for lentils or other beans you like.

RISOTTO WITH MUSHROOMS AND ASPARAGUS

GLUTEN-FREE
Serves 4
Prep time: 20 minutes
Pressure cook:
6 minutes high
pressure
**Pressure
release:** Quick
Total time: 45 to
50 minutes

PER SERVING: Calories: 480;
Fat: 11g; Carbohydrates: 77g;
Fiber: 4g; Sugar: 6g;
Protein: 16g; Sodium: 470mg

Risotto is a common Italian comfort food comprised of tender rice in a creamy sauce. There are a few short-grain varieties of rice that work best, but Arborio is my favorite. When making risotto, be sure to choose short-grain rice because the short, plump grains are best suited to absorb liquid, impart creaminess to the dish, maintain texture, and have a good bite.

1 tablespoon unsalted butter
1 tablespoon extra-virgin olive oil
8 ounces cremini mushrooms, thinly sliced
8 asparagus spears, thinly sliced
1 onion, finely diced
½ teaspoon kosher salt
¼ teaspoon freshly ground black pepper
3 tablespoons chopped fresh sage leaves
2 garlic cloves, minced
1½ cups Arborio rice
½ cup white wine
4 cups Vegetable Stock (page 140) or
   store-bought vegetable stock, warmed
½ cup grated Parmesan cheese

1. Press the sauté button on the Instant Pot, allow it to heat up, then drop in the butter and oil.

2. Once the butter has melted, add the mushrooms, asparagus, onion, salt, and pepper. Sauté, stirring occasionally, for about 8 minutes, or until softened.

3. Add the sage and garlic. Sauté for 30 seconds, or until fragrant.

4. Add the rice and sauté for 1 minute, or until starting to look translucent.

5. Add the wine and deglaze: Mix well and scrape up any brown bits on the bottom of the pot. Reduce the wine by half, about 1 minute.

6. Add the stock and mix well. Press the cancel button to stop cooking.

7. Secure the lid and cook on high pressure for 6 minutes.

8. After cooking, quick release the pressure. Unlock and remove the lid, then mix the risotto well. If liquid still remains, press the sauté button and cook, stirring continuously, until most of the liquid has been absorbed.

9. Add the cheese and mix well. Press the cancel button to stop cooking. Serve immediately.

SIMPLE SWAP: Risotto is a super versatile vegetarian option. Feel free to swap out the asparagus, mushrooms, and sage for other vegetables and herbs you like! You can also make this dairy-free by removing the cheese and swapping the butter for oil.

STUFFED SWEET POTATOES

GLUTEN-FREE
Serves 4
Prep time: 5 minutes
Pressure cook:
12 minutes high
pressure
**Pressure
release:** Quick
Total time: 25 to
30 minutes

PER SERVING: Calories: 290;
Fat: 5g; Carbohydrates: 52g;
Fiber: 10g; Sugar: 11g;
Protein: 12g; Sodium: 180mg

1 cup water
4 medium (6- to
  8-ounce) sweet
  potatoes
2 cups Basic Beans
  (page 135) or canned
  beans
1 cup Tzatziki
  (page 139)

Did you know there are more than 400 different varieties of sweet potatoes grown worldwide? They are all generally starchy and slightly sweet, but vary in shape, color, and texture, each with its own taste profile. They're all delicious and incredibly versatile, so grab your favorites and get these stuffed sweet potatoes going! A great addition to this dish is your favorite steamed or roasted vegetables.

1. Pour the water into the Instant Pot, and place the steam rack in the pot. Place the sweet potatoes on the steam rack. Secure the lid and cook on high pressure for 12 minutes.

2. After cooking, quick release the pressure. Unlock and remove the lid.

3. Carefully remove the sweet potatoes. Slice open lengthwise, and using a fork, fluff the inner flesh.

4. Stuff the sweet potatoes with the beans and tzatziki and serve.

SAVE FOR LATER: Making sweet potatoes in the Instant Pot is a great way to meal prep for the week. They can be served as a hearty vegetarian main dish, as this recipe shows, but they can also be integrated in other ways throughout the week.

SPAGHETTI SQUASH WITH CHERRY TOMATOES, BASIL, AND FETA

GLUTEN-FREE
Serves 4
Prep time: 15 minutes
Pressure cook:
10 minutes high
pressure
**Pressure
release:** Quick
Total time: 35 minutes

PER SERVING: Calories: 500;
Fat: 24g; Carbohydrates: 58g;
Fiber: 16g; Sugar: 14g;
Protein: 20g; Sodium: 350mg

1½ cups water
1 (3- to 3½-pound)
   spaghetti squash,
   halved and seeded
2 pints cherry
   tomatoes, halved
½ cup crumbled feta
   cheese
2 tablespoons
   extra-virgin olive oil
2 tablespoons freshly
   squeezed lemon juice
½ teaspoon kosher salt
¼ teaspoon freshly
   ground black pepper
⅓ cup pine nuts,
   toasted, for garnish
¼ cup fresh basil for
   garnish (optional)

Spaghetti squash is part of the winter squash family. It is typically large, yellow skinned, and oblong with a light-colored flesh that pulls away in strands resembling spaghetti when cooked. It is fairly neutral in flavor, has a tender and chewy texture, and is often used as a swap-in for pasta or grains. It is low in calories but is nutrient dense.

---

1. Pour the water into the Instant Pot, then add the squash, skin-side down and angled so as not to completely cover one half with the other half. Secure the lid and cook on high pressure for 10 minutes.

2. After cooking, quick release the pressure. Unlock and remove the lid.

3. Carefully transfer the squash to a cutting board. Using a fork, scrape the flesh out of the squash halves; it should come out easily and look similar to spaghetti.

4. In a large bowl, toss together the tomatoes, cheese, oil, lemon juice, salt, and pepper.

5. Add the squash strands to the bowl and toss.

6. Garnish with the pine nuts and basil (if using), and serve.

HELPFUL HACK: Sometimes large squash, like spaghetti squash, can be difficult to cut in half. To make the job easier, simply put the squash in the microwave and cook in 30-second intervals until you are able to cut it.

PASTA WITH MARINARA SAUCE

Serves 6
Prep time: 10 minutes
Pressure cook: 5 minutes high pressure
Pressure release: 5 minutes natural, then quick
Total time: 40 to 45 minutes

3 tablespoons extra-virgin olive oil
5 garlic cloves, sliced
1 (28-ounce) can low-sodium whole tomatoes, crushed with hands
1 tablespoon Italian seasoning
1 teaspoon honey
1 teaspoon kosher salt
¼ teaspoon freshly ground black pepper
1 pound rigatoni
2 cups Vegetable Stock (page 140) or store-bought vegetable stock
1½ cups water
½ cup grated Parmesan cheese, for garnish
½ cup fresh basil leaves, cut into ribbons, for garnish

This quick weeknight pasta with homemade sauce is sure to be a crowd-pleaser. To guarantee that the pasta does not overcook, the pressure cooking time is only 5 minutes. After the pressure is released, there's another 5 minutes, which allows the rigatoni to reach perfect al dente doneness.

1. Press the sauté button on the Instant Pot, allow it to heat up, then pour in the oil.

2. Add the garlic and sauté for about 30 seconds, or until fragrant.

3. Add the tomatoes with their juices, Italian seasoning, honey, salt, and pepper. Mix well. Simmer for about 5 minutes, or until thickened.

4. Stir in the rigatoni, stock, and water. Mix well, making sure all the rigatoni is submerged. Press the cancel button to stop cooking.

5. Secure the lid and cook on high pressure for 5 minutes.

6. After cooking, let the pressure release naturally for 5 minutes, then quick release the remaining pressure. Unlock and remove the lid, mix well, and let stand for 5 minutes.

7. Serve the pasta garnished with the cheese and basil.

PER SERVING: Calories: 415; Fat: 11g; Carbohydrates: 64g; Fiber: 4g; Sugar: 8g; Protein: 14g; Sodium: 375mg

SIMPLE SWAP: Any short, sturdy pasta will work in this recipe. Feel free to swap out the rigatoni for penne or ziti, for example.

JAMMY EGGS WITH HUMMUS AND RICE SALAD

DAIRY-FREE, GLUTEN-FREE

Serves 4
Prep time: 15 minutes
Total time: 15 minutes

PER SERVING: Calories: 375; Fat: 17g; Carbohydrates: 43g; Fiber: 8g; Sugar: 3g; Protein: 15g; Sodium: 290mg

1½ cups Hummus (page 138) or store-bought hummus

2 cups Basic Brown Rice (page 134)

8 cups mixed greens, such as arugula, baby spinach, green or red leaf lettuce

4 Soft-Boiled Eggs (page 136), peeled and halved

I love having a variety of flavors, textures, and types of food all in the same bowl. This delicious, simple dish provides all that you need in the form of creamy hummus, crisp greens, tender brown rice, and jammy soft-boiled eggs. For an extra boost of crunch, add your favorite toasted nuts as a topping. Perfect for a lunch break or light supper.

1. Spoon and spread out the hummus along the bottom of a large serving platter.

2. Top with the rice.

3. Scatter the greens on top.

4. Place the eggs on top and serve.

SIMPLE SWAP: Any type of whole grain works well in this dish. Feel free to swap out the brown rice for quinoa, farro, or black rice.

LENTIL RAGÙ

GLUTEN-FREE
Serves 6
Prep time: 10 minutes
Pressure cook:
15 minutes high
pressure
Pressure release:
15 minutes natural,
then quick
Total time: 55 minutes

PER SERVING: Calories: 250;
Fat: 3g; Carbohydrates: 42g;
Fiber: 18g; Sugar: 9g;
Protein: 14g; Sodium: 300mg

Looking for a plant-based alternative to a traditional Bolognese sauce, also known as vegan Bolognese? Look no further than this lentil ragù! Whether you are a vegetarian or not, this dish is a great way to sneak some more vegetables into your day. Perfect for a Meatless Monday or, let's face it, delicious any day of the week, this sauce goes great with Creamy Polenta with Crème Fraîche (page 42), or for an extra dose of veggies, serve it over zucchini noodles.

1 tablespoon extra-virgin olive oil
1 onion, diced
1 carrot, diced
1 teaspoon kosher salt
¼ teaspoon freshly ground black pepper
1 tablespoon dried basil
3 garlic cloves, minced
1 teaspoon dried thyme
1 teaspoon dried oregano
3 tablespoons tomato paste
3 cups Vegetable Stock (page 140) or
   store-bought vegetable stock
1 (15-ounce) can tomato sauce
1 (14½-ounce) can low-sodium diced tomatoes
1½ cups dried brown lentils
1 tablespoon red wine vinegar
½ cup chopped fresh basil leaves, for garnish

1. Press the sauté button on the Instant Pot, allow it to heat up, then pour in the oil.

2. Add the onion, carrot, salt, and pepper. Sauté for about 3 minutes, or until softened.

3. Add the basil, garlic, thyme, and oregano. Sauté for 30 seconds, or until fragrant.

4. Add the tomato paste and sauté for 1 minute.

5. Add the stock, tomato sauce, tomatoes with their juices, and lentils. Mix well. Press the cancel button to stop cooking.

6. Secure the lid and cook on high pressure for 15 minutes.

7. After cooking, let the pressure release naturally for 15 minutes, then quick release the remaining pressure. Unlock and remove the lid, and mix well.

8. Add the vinegar and mix well.

9. Serve the ragù garnished with the basil.

SAVE FOR LATER: Put any leftovers into an airtight container, and freeze. I recommend using appropriate portion-size containers so that you can thaw smaller quantities if needed. Don't forget to label the containers with the dish name and date!

COUSCOUS WITH EGGPLANT

**DAIRY-FREE,
Serves 4**
Prep time: 20 minutes
Pressure cook:
10 minutes high
pressure
**Pressure
release:** Quick
Total time: 50 minutes
to 1 hour

1 tablespoon
extra-virgin olive oil
1 onion, diced
1 tablespoon capers,
drained and rinsed
2 garlic cloves, minced
½ teaspoon kosher salt
¼ teaspoon freshly
ground black pepper
¼ teaspoon red pepper
flakes
1 eggplant, diced
(1 pound)
1 bunch kale, stemmed
and chopped
2 cups Vegetable
Stock (page 140)
or store-bought
vegetable stock
1¼ cups Israeli
couscous
2 oregano sprigs,
stemmed
2 thyme sprigs,
stemmed

Although couscous looks like a grain, it is actually a form of pasta. Couscous is made by rubbing semolina flour until tiny pieces are formed. Regular couscous is very small, whereas Israeli couscous is larger and similar to the size of a small pearl. This size gives more of a chewy bite to dishes compared to the smaller couscous variety.

1. Press the sauté button on the Instant Pot, allow it to heat up, then pour in the oil.

2. Add the onion and sauté for about 2 minutes, or until softened.

3. Add the capers, garlic, salt, pepper, and red pepper flakes. Sauté for about 30 seconds, or until fragrant.

4. Add the eggplant and sauté for about 3 minutes, or until softened.

5. Add the kale and cook, stirring, for about 1 minute, or until wilted.

6. Add the stock, couscous, oregano, and thyme. Mix together. Press the cancel button to stop cooking.

7. Secure the lid and cook on high pressure for 10 minutes.

8. After cooking, quick release the pressure. Unlock and remove the lid, mix well, and let stand for 5 to 10 minutes. Serve warm.

HELPFUL HACK: Be sure to dice the eggplant into ½- to 1-inch pieces and chop or tear the kale into small pieces. This makes it easier to cook and eat.

PER SERVING: Calories: 345; Fat: 5g; Carbohydrates: 71g; Fiber: 9g; Sugar: 10g; Protein: 14g; Sodium: 285mg

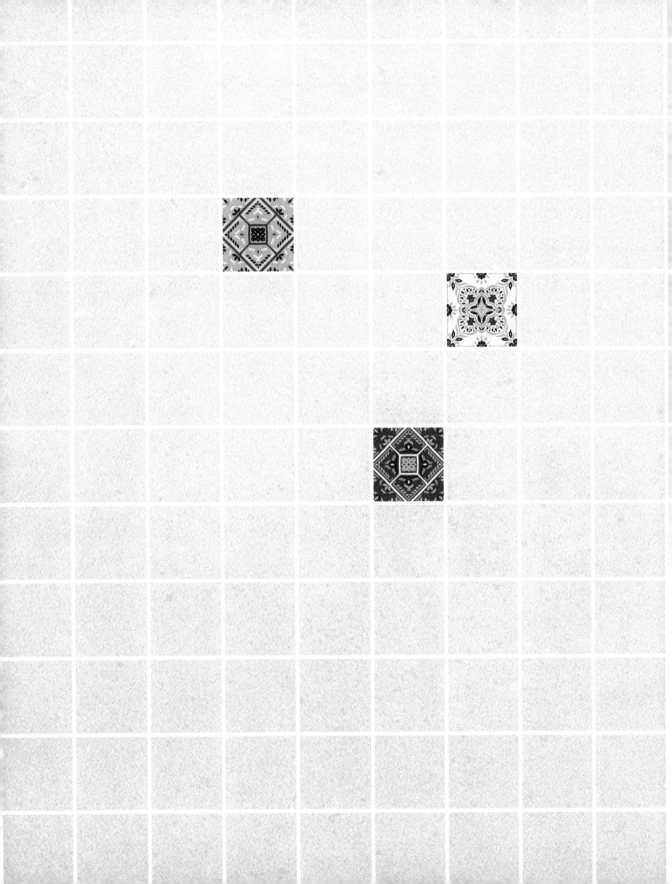

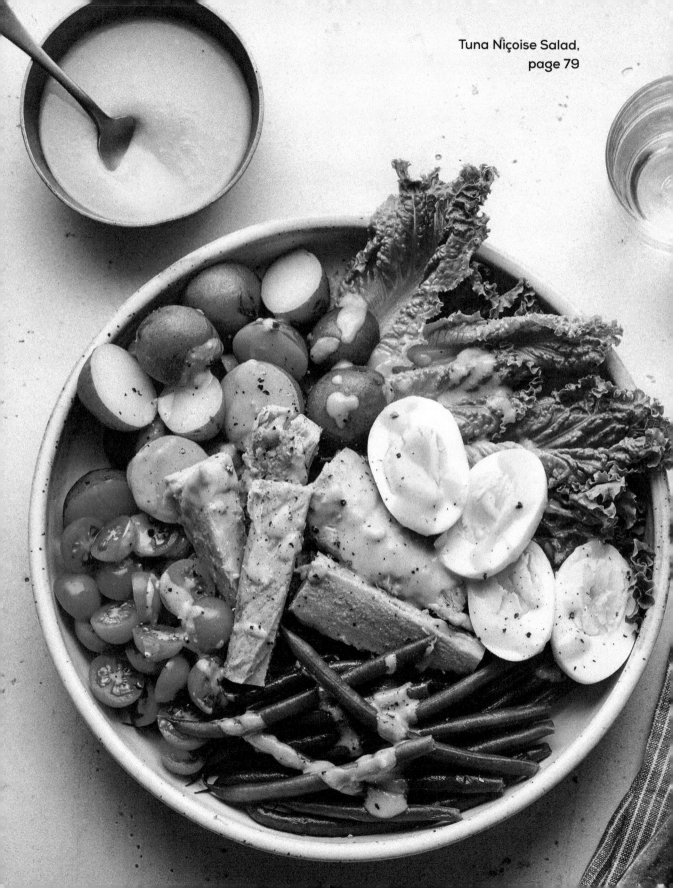

Tuna Niçoise Salad,
page 79

CHAPTER SIX

SEAFOOD

Mussels with Harissa. 76

Cold-Poached Salmon Salad 78

Tuna Niçoise Salad 79

Shrimp with Lentils 80

Halibut with Tomato-Chile Sauce 82

Poached Shrimp with Mediterranean "Cocktail Sauce" 85

Monkfish with Kale and White Beans 86

Cod with Puttanesca. 88

Steamed Clams 89

Salmon with Basil-Walnut Pesto. 90

Whole Branzino 91

MUSSELS WITH HARISSA

**DAIRY-FREE,
GLUTEN-FREE**

Serves 2

Prep time: 15 minutes

Pressure cook:
2 minutes high
pressure

**Pressure
release:** Quick

Total time: 30 minutes

PER SERVING: Calories: 300;
Fat: 12g; Carbohydrates: 16g;
Fiber: 3g; Sugar: 3g;
Protein: 29g; Sodium: 900mg

2 tablespoons
   extra-virgin olive oil
1 shallot, diced
1 cup Vegetable
   Stock (page 140)
   or store-bought
   vegetable stock
1 tablespoon harissa
1 (14-ounce) can
   artichoke hearts,
   drained and rinsed
1 cup diced bell pepper
2 pounds mussels,
   scrubbed and
   debearded
2 tablespoons
   chopped fresh
   parsley, for garnish
Crusty bread, for serving

Harissa is a spicy, aromatic, and flavorful pepper or chili paste that is widely used in Mediterranean cooking. It may vary depending on the country, but it is generally a blend of hot chile peppers, olive oil, garlic, and spices. It may range from mild to hot, so be sure to choose whichever you prefer. It is most commonly found in ready-made jars, tubes, or cans in the grocery store.

1. Press the sauté button on the Instant Pot, allow it to heat up, then pour in the oil.

2. Add the shallot and sauté for 3 minutes, or until softened.

3. Add the stock and harissa. Deglaze: Mix well and scrape up any brown bits on the bottom of the pot.

4. Add the artichoke hearts and bell pepper. Mix well.

5. Add the mussels. Press the cancel button to stop cooking.

6. Secure the lid and cook on high pressure for 2 minutes.

7. After cooking, quick release the pressure. Unlock and remove the lid.

8. Transfer the mussels to a large serving bowl.

9. Garnish with the parsley, and serve with crusty bread.

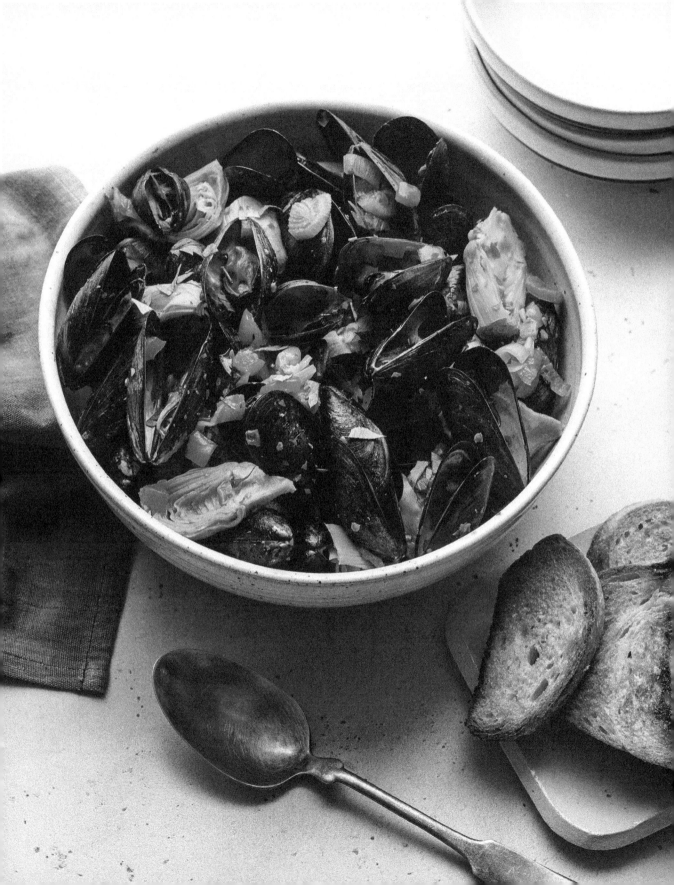

COLD-POACHED SALMON SALAD

DAIRY-FREE, GLUTEN-FREE

Serves 2
Prep time: 15 minutes
Pressure cook:
4 minutes low pressure
Pressure release: Quick
Total time: 30 to
35 minutes, plus 1 hour
to chill

1½ cups Vegetable
   Stock (page 140)
   or store-bought
   vegetable stock
½ cup white wine
1 lemon, thinly sliced
1 bay leaf
Olive oil cooking spray,
   for coating the steam
   rack
2 (6-ounce) salmon
   fillets
½ teaspoon kosher salt
¼ teaspoon freshly
   ground black pepper
1 head Boston or Bibb
   lettuce
1 cup sliced radishes
1 cup cherry tomatoes,
   halved
¼ cup Tahini Dressing
   (page 144)

This poached salmon dish is a delicious lunch or light dinner. Salmon characteristics may vary with the species, ranging in color from orange to pink or red. Widely known as an excellent source of brain-boosting omega-3 fatty acids, salmon is also rich in protein, potassium, selenium, and vitamin B_{12}.

1. In the Instant Pot, combine the stock, wine, lemon, and bay leaf.

2. Coat a steam rack with cooking spray and put it inside the pot, handles extending up. Place the salmon fillets, skin-side down, on the prepared steam rack. Season with the salt and pepper.

3. Secure the lid and cook on low pressure for 4 minutes.

4. After cooking, quick release the pressure. Unlock and remove the lid.

5. Carefully remove the inner pot, and let sit at room temperature for 10 minutes. Then refrigerate for 1 hour.

6. Split the lettuce between 2 large plates.

7. Divide the salmon fillets, radishes, and tomatoes between the plates.

8. Drizzle with the dressing and serve.

PER SERVING: Calories: 470; Fat: 32g; Carbohydrates: 7g; Fiber: 3g; Sugar: 3g; Protein: 38g; Sodium: 550mg

SAVE FOR LATER: Salmon can be cooked ahead and kept in the refrigerator up to 24 hours prior to serving.

TUNA NIÇOISE SALAD

**DAIRY-FREE,
GLUTEN-FREE**

Serves 2

Prep time: 20 minutes

Pressure cook:
3 minutes high
pressure

**Pressure
release:** Quick

Total time: 30 to
35 minutes

PER SERVING:
Calories: 600; Fat: 32g;
Carbohydrates: 42g;
Fiber: 13g; Sugar: 12g;
Protein: 44g; Sodium: 465mg

**FOR THE POTATOES,
GREEN BEANS,
AND EGGS**

1 cup water

8 ounces mini
   potatoes, halved

8 ounces green beans,
   trimmed

2 large eggs

FOR THE SALAD

1 head romaine lettuce,
   chopped

1 cup cherry tomatoes,
   halved

1 (7-ounce) jar
   oil-packed tuna,
   drained

¼ cup Tahini Dressing
   (page 144)

Tuna Niçoise salad originated in France in the city of Nice. It is often prepared as a composed salad, meaning there is romaine across the bottom, but each remaining ingredient is placed in its own area on top of the greens. Some versions also contain anchovies or Niçoise olives, which would make a delicious addition to this recipe as well.

**TO MAKE THE POTATOES, GREEN BEANS,
AND EGGS**

1. Fill a large bowl with ice water and set aside.

2. Pour the water into the Instant Pot. Place the potatoes, green beans, and eggs in a steamer basket. Gently place in the pot. Secure the lid and cook on high pressure for 3 minutes.

3. After cooking, quick release the pressure. Unlock and remove the lid.

4. Transfer the vegetables and eggs to the ice water bath.

5. Peel and halve the eggs.

TO MAKE THE SALAD

6. While everything is cooking, arrange the lettuce on a serving platter.

7. Place the tomatoes, eggs, green beans, potatoes, and tuna on top.

8. Serve the salad topped with the dressing.

SIMPLE SWAP: Feel free to use whatever dressing you like. A simple mix of oil and vinegar is always great!

SHRIMP WITH LENTILS

**DAIRY-FREE,
GLUTEN-FREE**

Serves 4
Prep time: 20 minutes
Pressure cook:
20 minutes high
pressure
Pressure release:
10 minutes natural,
then quick
Total time: 1 hour
10 minutes

PER SERVING: Calories: 365;
Fat: 7g; Carbohydrates: 43g;
Fiber: 11g; Sugar: 9g;
Protein: 35g; Sodium: 555mg

This hearty meal provides a full range of healthy fats, lean protein, and complex carbohydrates—and it's easy to make and tastes delicious. Lentils are an affordable legume, providing dietary fiber and complex carbohydrates as well as vitamins and minerals, such as folate and manganese. Shrimp is an excellent source of lean protein, zinc, and magnesium. Rounding out the dish is an assortment of vegetables, providing even more nutrients.

1 tablespoon extra-virgin olive oil
1 onion, diced
1 carrot, diced
1 bell pepper, diced
3 garlic cloves, minced
1 teaspoon kosher salt
1 tablespoon sweet paprika
¼ teaspoon red pepper flakes
1 pound plum tomatoes, chopped
2½ cups Vegetable Stock (page 140) or
    store-bought vegetable stock
1 cup dried French green lentils
1 pound shrimp, peeled and deveined
Juice of 1 lemon
1 tablespoon tahini (optional)

1. Press the sauté button on the Instant Pot, allow it to heat up, then pour in the oil.

2. Add the onion, carrot, and bell pepper. Sauté for 3 minutes, or until softened.

3. Add the garlic, salt, paprika, and red pepper flakes. Sauté for 30 seconds, or until fragrant.

4. Add the tomatoes, stock, and lentils. Mix well. Press the cancel button to stop cooking.

5. Secure the lid and cook on high pressure for 20 minutes.

6. After cooking, let the pressure release naturally for 10 minutes, then quick release the remaining pressure. Unlock and remove the lid, then mix well.

7. Add the shrimp, and place the lid askew over the pot. Press the sauté button and simmer for about 4 minutes, or until the shrimp has cooked through. Press the cancel button to stop cooking.

8. Add the lemon juice and mix well.

9. Serve the shrimp and lentils drizzled with the tahini (if using).

SIMPLE SWAP: Feel free to swap out the plum tomatoes for 1 (14½-ounce) can of diced tomatoes. The stock can also be replaced with water.

HALIBUT WITH TOMATO-CHILE SAUCE

**DAIRY-FREE,
GLUTEN-FREE**

Serves 4
Prep time: 15 minutes
Pressure cook:
2 minutes high
pressure
**Pressure
release:** Quick
Total time: 40 to
45 minutes

PER SERVING:
Calories: 340; Fat: 15g;
Carbohydrates: 13g; Fiber:
4g; Sugar: 8g;
Protein: 39g; Sodium: 420mg

SIMPLE SWAP: This
recipe works well with
any hearty white fish.
Feel free to swap out
the halibut for whatever
you prefer, such as cod
or bass.

The fiery tomato-chile sauce in this dish pairs well with a hearty white fish like halibut; the added touch of rich tahini at the end helps counter some of the heat. It also tastes scrumptious on top of roasted poultry or mixed in with whole grains.

---

2 tablespoons extra-virgin olive oil
1 jalapeño or red chile, seeded and finely diced
4 garlic cloves, sliced
1½ pounds plum tomatoes, diced
1 poblano pepper, seeded and diced
3 tablespoons tomato paste
1 teaspoon kosher salt
1 teaspoon ground cumin
½ teaspoon honey
½ cup water, Vegetable Stock (page 140), or
   store-bought vegetable stock
4 (6-ounce) halibut fillets
¼ cup chopped fresh cilantro, for garnish
2 tablespoons tahini

1. Press the sauté button on the Instant Pot, allow it to heat up, then pour in the oil.

2. Add the jalapeño and sauté for 1 minute.

3. Add the garlic and sauté for 30 seconds, or until fragrant.

4. Add the tomatoes and poblano pepper. Cook for 3 minutes, or until softened.

5. Add the tomato paste, salt, cumin, and honey. Sauté for 1 minute.

6. Add the water and deglaze: Mix well and scrape up any brown bits on the bottom of the pot. Press the cancel button to stop cooking.

7. Secure the lid and cook on high pressure for 2 minutes.

8. After cooking, quick release the pressure. Unlock and remove the lid, then mix well.

9. Nestle the halibut fillets into the mixture. Press the sauté button, place the lid askew over the pot, and simmer for 10 to 12 minutes, or until the halibut is cooked through and opaque. Press the cancel button to stop cooking.

10. Serve the halibut garnished with the cilantro and drizzled with the tahini.

SAVE FOR LATER: The sauce can be batched up and saved for a future use. Simply remove half after step 7, put in an airtight container, and freeze for up to 6 months.

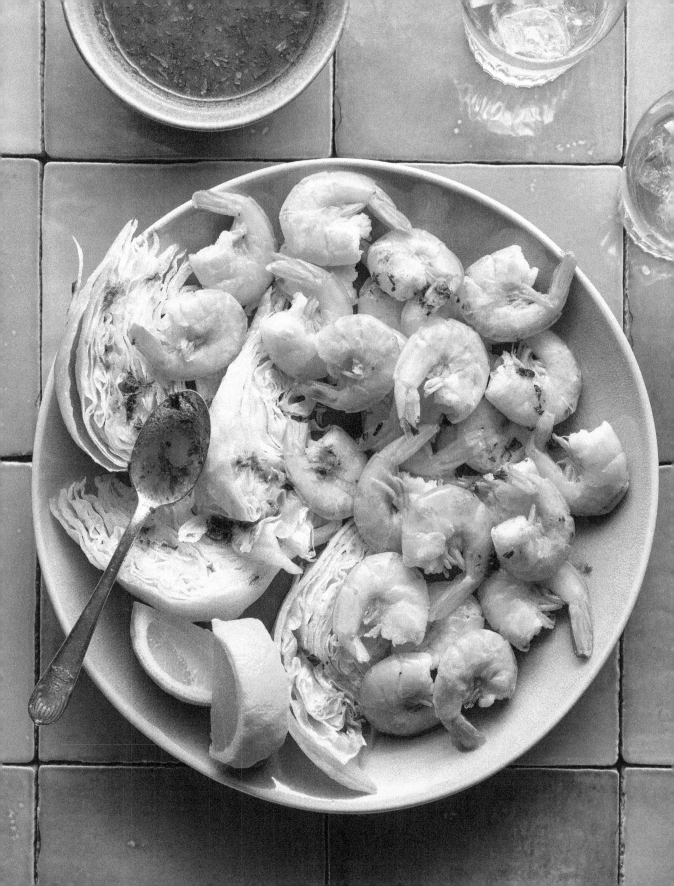

POACHED SHRIMP WITH MEDITERRANEAN "COCKTAIL SAUCE"

DAIRY-FREE, GLUTEN-FREE

Serves 4
Prep time: 5 minutes
Pressure cook: 1 minute low pressure
Pressure release: 10 minutes natural, then quick
Total time: 20 to 25 minutes

PER SERVING: Calories: 130; Fat: 3g; Carbohydrates: 3g; Fiber: 0g; Sugar: 0g; Protein: 23g; Sodium: 235mg

FOR THE SHRIMP
1 pound large frozen shrimp
2 cups water
1 teaspoon kosher salt

FOR THE COCKTAIL SAUCE
¼ cup water
¼ cup harissa
¼ cup chopped fresh mint leaves
Juice of ½ lemon

I love this recipe because it is super quick and uses shrimp straight from the freezer. For best results, choose EZ-peel shrimp that are large, so 31 to 40 per pound. The poached shrimp is meant to be served cold, but it will be just as delicious if you skip the ice bath in step 4 and serve it warm.

TO MAKE THE SHRIMP

1. Fill a medium bowl with ice water and set aside.

2. In the Instant Pot, combine the shrimp, water, and salt. Mix well. Secure the lid and cook on low pressure for 1 minute.

3. After cooking, let the pressure release naturally for 10 minutes, then quick release the remaining pressure. Unlock and remove the lid.

4. Drain the shrimp in a colander, then immediately place in the ice water bath to stop cooking.

TO MAKE THE COCKTAIL SAUCE

5. While the shrimp is cooking, in a small bowl, mix together the water, harissa, mint, and lemon juice.

6. Serve the shrimp with the cocktail sauce on the side.

SIMPLE SWAP: If you don't want to use this Mediterranean version of cocktail sauce, try pairing the shrimp with Basil-Walnut Pesto (page 142) or with any sauce you like.

MONKFISH WITH KALE AND WHITE BEANS

DAIRY-FREE, GLUTEN-FREE

Serves 4
Prep time: 15 minutes
Pressure cook:
5 minutes high pressure
Pressure release:
10 minutes natural, then quick
Total time: 45 minutes

PER SERVING: Calories: 330; Fat: 9g; Carbohydrates: 30g; Fiber: 8g; Sugar: 3g; Protein: 27g; Sodium: 270mg

Monkfish has often been called the "poor man's lobster" and can be found across the Mediterranean Sea, particularly along the coast of Europe. It has a mild, slightly sweet taste and is dense, firm, and boneless, similar to lobster tail. Its firm texture means that it will not fall apart when cooked, so it typically holds up very well in the Instant Pot.

2 tablespoons extra-virgin olive oil
1 onion, diced
1 tablespoon minced fresh rosemary leaves
2 garlic cloves, minced
¾ teaspoon kosher salt
¼ teaspoon red pepper flakes
1 bunch kale, stemmed and chopped
2 cups Basic Beans (page 135) or canned cannellini beans
½ cup white wine
½ cup Vegetable Stock (page 140) or store-bought vegetable stock
1 pound monkfish
Juice of ½ lemon

1. Press the sauté button on the Instant Pot, allow it to heat up, then pour in the oil.

2. Add the onion and sauté for 2 minutes, or until softened.

3. Add the rosemary, garlic, salt, and red pepper flakes. Sauté for 30 seconds, or until fragrant.

4. Add the kale and sauté for 2 minutes, or until wilted.

5. Add the beans and sauté for 1 minute.

6. Add the wine and deglaze: Mix well and scrape up any brown bits on the bottom of the pot.

7. Add the stock and mix well.

8. Nestle the monkfish in the pot. Press the cancel button to stop cooking.

9. Secure the lid and cook on high pressure for 5 minutes.

10. After cooking, let the pressure release naturally for 10 minutes, then quick release the remaining pressure. Unlock and remove the lid, then mix well. The fish should be cooked through and opaque. If it is not quite cooked through, press the sauté button, place the lid askew over the pot, and simmer until finished. Press the cancel button to stop cooking.

11. Add the lemon juice, mix well, and serve.

HELPFUL HACK: Pre-packaged chopped kale or baby kale can be used in place of the regular bunch of kale, which may cut down on prep time. Other greens, such as Swiss chard or spinach, may be used in place of the kale as well.

COD WITH PUTTANESCA

**DAIRY-FREE,
GLUTEN-FREE**

Serves 4
Prep time: 15 minutes
Pressure cook:
3 minutes high
pressure
**Pressure
release:** Quick
Total time: 35 to
40 minutes

PER SERVING: Calories:
225; Fat: 6g; Carbohydrates:
10g; Fiber: 2g; Sugar: 5g;
Protein: 32g; Sodium: 540mg

---

1 tablespoon
   extra-virgin olive oil
3 garlic cloves, minced
1 tablespoon tomato
   paste
1 teaspoon anchovy
   paste
½ teaspoon kosher salt
¼ teaspoon red pepper
   flakes
1 (28-ounce) can
   low-sodium whole
   tomatoes, crushed
½ cup water
⅓ cup chopped fresh
   basil leaves
⅓ cup chopped pitted
   Kalamata olives
1 tablespoon capers,
   drained and rinsed
4 (6-ounce) cod fillets

Puttanesca is a sauce composed of capers and olives. It is typically tossed with pasta; however, it pairs beautifully with hearty white fish like cod. I've added some anchovy paste for an extra briny kick, but you can remove that completely or replace it with some chopped jarred anchovies. The heat can be eased up or kicked up a notch by adjusting the amount of red pepper flakes.

1. Press the sauté function on the Instant Pot, allow it to heat up, then pour in the oil.

2. Add the garlic and sauté for 30 seconds, or until fragrant.

3. Add the tomato paste, anchovy paste, salt, and red pepper flakes. Sauté for 30 seconds.

4. Add the tomatoes with their juices, water, basil, olives, and capers. Mix well. Press the cancel button to stop cooking.

5. Secure the lid and cook on high pressure for 3 minutes.

6. After cooking, quick release the pressure. Unlock and remove the lid, then mix well.

7. Add the cod fillets, and place the lid askew over the pot. Press the sauté button and simmer for about 10 minutes, or until the cod is cooked through and opaque. Press the cancel button to stop cooking.

8. If desired, garnish with fresh parsley and serve.

SIMPLE SWAP: Any type of fish fillets you like should work well in place of the cod fillets.

STEAMED CLAMS

**DAIRY-FREE,
GLUTEN-FREE**

Serves 2
Prep time: 10 minutes
Pressure cook:
4 minutes high
pressure
Pressure release:
15 minutes natural,
then quick
Total time: 40 to
45 minutes

PER SERVING: Calories: 340;
Fat: 4g; Carbohydrates: 13g;
Fiber: 1g; Sugar: 1g;
Protein: 58g; Sodium: 320mg

**2 pounds littleneck
clams, washed and
scrubbed**
**½ cup Vegetable
Stock (page 140)
or store-bought
vegetable stock**
½ cup white wine
**2 tablespoons
chopped fresh basil
leaves**
**1 tablespoon
extra-virgin olive oil**
**1 tablespoon freshly
squeezed lemon juice**
**Crusty bread, for
serving**

Steamed Clams are an easy, delicious dinner if you're in the mood for a pot of seafood. Clam shells can be fairly sandy, so be sure to scrub them well with a plastic brush prior to cooking. Some shells may not open initially, or at all. Be sure to follow the instructions on what to do in this event.

1. In the Instant Pot, combine the clams, stock, wine, basil, oil, and lemon juice. Secure the lid and cook on high pressure for 4 minutes.

2. After cooking, let the pressure release naturally for 15 minutes, then quick release the remaining pressure. Unlock and remove the lid. If some clams are still closed, press the sauté button, and simmer for 1 to 2 minutes. Press the cancel button to stop cooking. Discard any unopened clams. Transfer to a serving dish.

3. Serve the clams with crusty bread.

SIMPLE SWAP: If you cannot find littleneck clams or simply prefer a different type, any clams will work well with this recipe.

SALMON WITH BASIL-WALNUT PESTO

GLUTEN-FREE
Serves 4
Prep time: 5 minutes
Pressure cook:
3 minutes low pressure
Pressure release: Quick
Total time: 10 to 15 minutes

PER SERVING: Calories: 400; Fat: 29g; Carbohydrates: 1g; Fiber: 0g; Sugar: 0g; Protein: 33g; Sodium: 320mg

---

½ cup Vegetable Stock (page 140) or store-bought vegetable stock

½ cup loosely packed fresh parsley

Olive oil cooking spray, for coating the steam rack

1⅓ pounds salmon fillets, about 1 inch thick

½ teaspoon kosher salt

¼ teaspoon freshly ground black pepper

¼ cup Basil-Walnut Pesto (page 142) or store-bought pesto

These salmon fillets are topped with tasty Basil-Walnut Pesto, which is an easy and delicious way to get those heart-healthy omega-3 fatty acids! If you prefer to have individual portions prepped prior to cooking, simply cut the salmon fillet into four pieces or purchase four separate 5-ounce portions. Serve with Basic Brown Rice (page 134) or Greek-Style Lentils (page 46).

1. In the Instant Pot, combine the stock and parsley.

2. Coat the steam rack with cooking spray and put it inside the pot, handles extending up. Place the salmon, skin-side down, on the prepared steam rack. Season with the salt and pepper.

3. Secure the lid and cook on low pressure for 3 minutes.

4. After cooking, quick release the pressure. Unlock and remove the lid.

5. Carefully remove the steam rack with the salmon.

6. Cut the salmon into 4 portions.

7. Top each portion with 1 tablespoon of pesto.

SIMPLE SWAP: Not a fan of salmon or simply looking to try a different variety of fish? Arctic char and cod are both great options.

WHOLE BRANZINO

DAIRY-FREE, GLUTEN-FREE

Serves 2

Prep time: 5 minutes
Pressure cook: 7 minutes high pressure
Pressure release: Quick
Total time: 20 to 25 minutes

PER SERVING: Calories: 220; Fat: 7g; Carbohydrates: 0g; Fiber: 0g; Sugar: 0g; Protein: 36g; Sodium: 365mg

---

1 whole branzino, cleaned and scaled
½ teaspoon kosher salt
¼ teaspoon freshly ground black pepper
1 cup water
Olive oil cooking spray, for coating the steam rack
1 lemon, thinly sliced

Branzino has been called European bass and is very popular in Mediterranean cuisine. Cooking and serving a whole fish doesn't have to be reserved for restaurant meals! This simple, tasty, and healthy recipe can easily be made any day of the week. To round out the meal, serve it with Farro with Herby Yogurt (page 48).

---

1. Season the inside of the branzino with the salt and pepper.

2. Pour the water into the Instant Pot.

3. Coat a steam rack with cooking spray and put it inside the pot, handles extending up. Place the branzino on the prepared steam rack.

4. Place half of the lemon slices on top of the fish.

5. Secure the lid and cook on high pressure for 7 minutes.

6. After cooking, quick release the pressure. Unlock and remove the lid.

7. Carefully remove the steam rack with the branzino.

8. Place the branzino on a serving platter with the remaining lemon slices. Remove the fillets; they should easily separate and pull away from the bones. Serve immediately.

SIMPLE SWAP: Any whole fish or large side of fish or fillet that can fit in your Instant Pot would work well with this recipe. Just be sure the fish you choose has been cleaned and scaled.

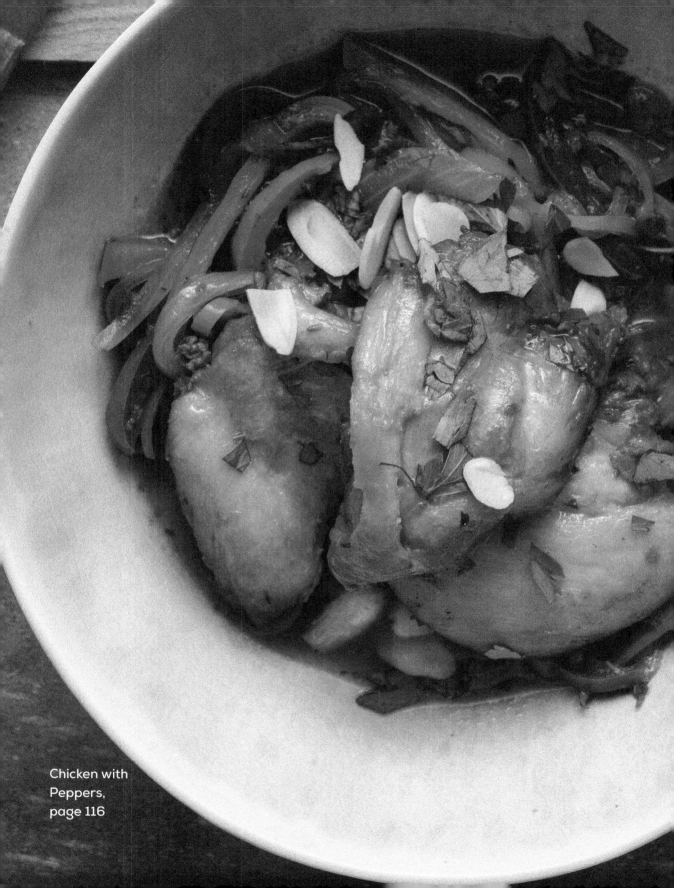

Chicken with
Peppers,
page 116

CHAPTER SEVEN

POULTRY AND MEAT

Sausage-Bean Soup 94

Avgolemono (Greek Chicken and Egg Soup) 95

Osso Buco 97

Shredded Chicken with Harissa 99

Mediterranean-Style Brisket .100

Moroccan Lamb 102

Whole Chicken 104

Green Chicken Soup 105

Lemon Chicken with Rosemary 106

Deconstructed Lamb-Stuffed Cabbage 107

Lamb Meat Loaf with Tahini Sauce 108

Braised Chicken with Tomato and Olives 111

Chicken with Mushrooms 113

Pork Ragù 114

Chicken with Peppers 116

SAUSAGE-BEAN SOUP

**DAIRY-FREE,
GLUTEN-FREE**

Serves 6
Prep time: 20 minutes
Pressure cook:
30 minutes high
pressure
Pressure release:
20 minutes natural,
then quick
Total time: 1 hour
30 minutes

2 tablespoons
  vegetable oil, divided
1 pound sausage
1 onion, diced
1 carrot, diced
1 celery stalk, diced
2 garlic cloves, minced
¾ teaspoon kosher salt
½ teaspoon dried
  thyme
½ teaspoon dried sage
¼ teaspoon freshly
  ground black pepper
4 cups Chicken
  Stock (page 141)
  or store-bought
  gluten-free chicken
  stock
1½ cups dried kidney
  beans
1 bay leaf
Juice of 1 lemon
Pita or crusty bread,
  for serving

Browning the sausage adds a flavorful depth
to the finished dish. Cooking the sausage whole
before slicing helps keep its texture intact, a wel-
come addition to this delicious soup. To ramp up
the vegetables, mix in some chopped spinach or
Swiss chard at the end with the lemon juice.

1. Press the sauté button on the Instant Pot, allow it
   to heat up, then pour in 1 tablespoon of oil.

2. Add the sausage and cook, turning, for about
   3 minutes, or until brown on all sides. Transfer to
   a cutting board. Cut into bite-size rounds.

3. Add the remaining 1 tablespoon of oil, the onion,
   carrot, and celery to the pot. Sauté for 3 minutes,
   or until the vegetables start to soften.

4. Add the garlic, salt, thyme, sage, and pepper. Sauté
   for 30 seconds, or until fragrant.

5. Add the stock, beans, bay leaf, and sausage. Press
   the cancel button to stop cooking.

6. Secure the lid and cook on high pressure for
   30 minutes.

7. After cooking, let the pressure release naturally
   for 20 minutes, then quick release the remaining
   pressure. Unlock and remove the lid.

8. Add the lemon juice and mix well.

9. Serve the soup warm with some pita or
   crusty bread.

PER SERVING: Calories: 330; Fat: 11g; Carbohydrates: 34g;
Fiber: 12g; Sugar: 3g; Protein: 25g; Sodium: 990mg

SIMPLE SWAP: Switch up the kidney beans with
another dried bean, or the flavor of sausage.

AVGOLEMONO (GREEK CHICKEN AND EGG SOUP)

**DAIRY-FREE,
GLUTEN-FREE**

Serves 6
Prep time: 15 minutes
Pressure cook:
15 minutes high
pressure
**Pressure
release:** Quick
Total time: 40 to
45 minutes

4 cups Chicken
   Stock (page 141)
   or store-bought
   gluten-free chicken
   stock
1 pound boneless,
   skinless chicken
   breasts
¾ teaspoon kosher salt
½ teaspoon dried
   thyme
½ teaspoon dried
   oregano
¼ teaspoon freshly
   ground black pepper
2 cups Basic Brown
   Rice (page 134),
   divided
3 tablespoons freshly
   squeezed lemon juice
2 large egg yolks
2 tablespoons
   chopped fresh dill, for
   garnish

Avgolemono is basically a Greek version of chicken and rice soup that is thickened with egg yolks. It is a bright, light dish that is perfect for a lunch or low-key dinner. Drizzle with extra-virgin olive oil before serving.

1. In the Instant Pot, combine the stock, chicken, salt, thyme, oregano, and pepper. Mix well. Secure the lid and cook on high pressure for 15 minutes.

2. After cooking, quick release the pressure. Unlock and remove the lid.

3. Transfer the chicken to a cutting board. Shred using 2 forks.

4. In a blender, process ½ cup of rice, the lemon juice, and egg yolks.

5. Slowly add 1 cup of the hot broth from the Instant Pot and continue to process.

6. Add the mixture to the Instant Pot along with the shredded chicken and remaining 1½ cups of brown rice.

7. Press the sauté button and simmer for 5 minutes, or until the soup has thickened. Press the cancel button to stop cooking.

8. Garnish the soup with dill before serving.

PER SERVING: Calories: 190; Fat: 4g; Carbohydrates: 16g; Fiber: 1g; Sugar: 1g; Protein: 21g; Sodium: 580mg

TROUBLESHOOTING TIP: The egg yolk mixture is meant to thicken the soup. If the soup does not thicken after 5 minutes of simmering in step 7, continue to simmer for another 5 minutes, stirring occasionally.

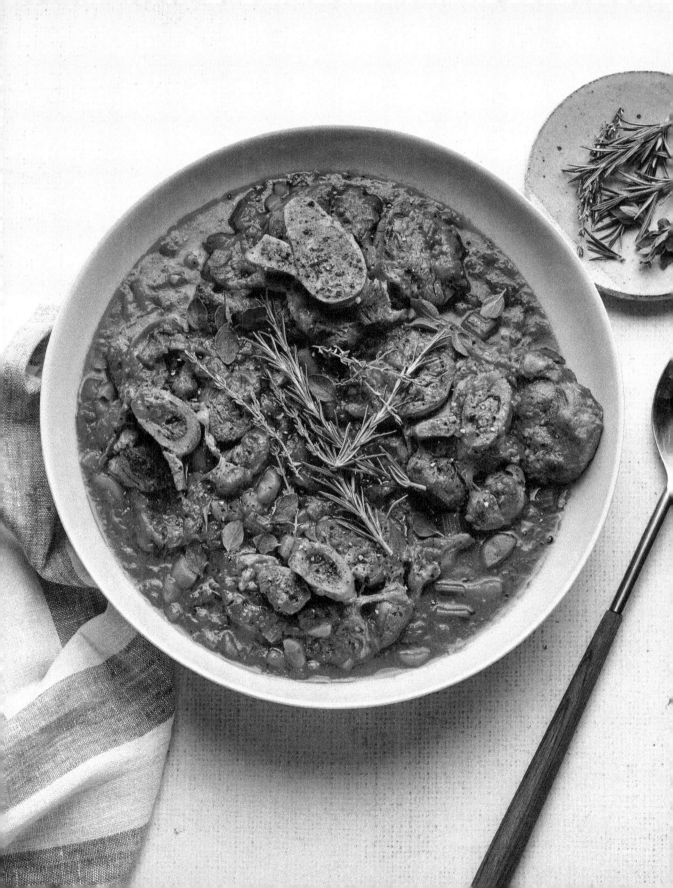

OSSO BUCO

DAIRY-FREE
Serves 4
Prep time: 15 minutes
Pressure cook:
40 minutes high
pressure
Pressure release:
20 minutes natural,
then quick
Total time: 2 hours
5 minutes

PER SERVING: Calories: 490;
Fat: 17g; Carbohydrates: 31g;
Fiber: 5g; Sugar: 10g;
Protein: 49g; Sodium: 600mg

Osso buco is a classic braised veal dish from northern Italy whose name literally translates to "bone with a hole." The cut of veal used has a round, marrow-filled bone that is a special treat. Be sure to grab a small spoon to try that silky bone marrow on a piece of crusty bread. This delicious, hearty meal tastes amazing when it's made and even better the next day! Pair it with Basic Brown Rice (page 134) to round out the meal, and garnish with fresh herbs if desired.

2 to 2½ pounds osso buco (4 pieces)
1 teaspoon kosher salt
½ teaspoon freshly ground black pepper
½ cup all-purpose flour
3 tablespoons extra-virgin olive oil, divided
3 carrots, diced
1 onion, diced
2 celery stalks, diced
5 garlic cloves, sliced
1 tablespoon tomato paste
½ cup red wine
1 (28-ounce) can low-sodium whole tomatoes
½ cup beef stock
4 thyme sprigs
2 rosemary sprigs
1 oregano sprig
1 bay leaf

1. Season the osso buco all over with the salt and pepper and dredge it in the flour.

2. Press the sauté button on the Instant Pot, allow it to heat up, then pour in 2 tablespoons of oil.

continued ➤

3. Add the osso buco and cook for about 5 minutes per side, or until browned all over. Remove the osso buco and set aside.

4. In the Instant Pot, combine the carrots, onion, celery, and remaining 1 tablespoon of oil. Sauté for 8 minutes, or until softened.

5. Add the garlic and tomato paste. Sauté for 30 seconds, or until fragrant.

6. Add the wine and deglaze: Mix well and scrape up any brown bits on the bottom of the pot.

7. Add the tomatoes with their juices, stock, thyme, rosemary, oregano, and bay leaf. Mix well.

8. Nestle the osso buco into the mixture. Press the cancel button to stop cooking.

9. Secure the lid and cook on high pressure for 40 minutes.

10. After cooking, let the pressure release naturally for 20 minutes, then quick release the remaining pressure. Unlock and remove the lid.

11. Carefully remove the herb sprigs and osso buco and set aside.

12. Press the sauté button and simmer the sauce for at least 10 minutes, or until reduced to your desired consistency. Press the cancel button to stop cooking.

13. Return the osso buco to the pot and serve.

SIMPLE SWAP: Dried herbs can be used in place of the fresh: Simply use ¼ teaspoon of oregano, ½ teaspoon of thyme, and ½ teaspoon of rosemary.

SHREDDED CHICKEN WITH HARISSA

**DAIRY-FREE,
GLUTEN-FREE**

Serves 4
Prep time: 10 minutes
Pressure cook:
25 minutes high
pressure
Pressure release:
20 minutes natural,
then quick
Total time: 1 hour
5 minutes

PER SERVING: Calories: 150;
Fat: 4g; Carbohydrates: 2g;
Fiber: 0g; Sugar: 0g;
Protein: 26g; Sodium: 425mg

1 pound boneless,
   skinless chicken
   breasts
1 cup Chicken
   Stock (page 141)
   or store-bought
   gluten-free chicken
   stock
⅓ cup harissa
½ teaspoon kosher salt
¼ teaspoon freshly
   ground black pepper

Harissa is a flavorful, aromatic chile pepper paste or sauce that is widely used in some Mediterranean regions, specifically North African and Middle Eastern countries. This recipe can be mild, medium, or spicy, depending on the harissa you choose. Pair with Tzatziki (page 139) for a refreshing combination that is sure to delight.

1. In the Instant Pot, combine the chicken, stock, harissa, salt, and pepper. Mix well. Secure the lid and cook on high pressure for 25 minutes.

2. After cooking, let the pressure release naturally for 20 minutes, then quick release the remaining pressure. Unlock and remove the lid.

3. Using 2 forks, shred the chicken. Serve immediately.

SIMPLE SWAP: Boneless, skinless chicken thighs can be used in place of the chicken breasts.

MEDITERRANEAN-STYLE BRISKET

**DAIRY-FREE,
GLUTEN-FREE**

Serves 8

Prep time: 1 hour

Pressure cook:
1 hour 15 minutes high
pressure

Pressure release:
30 minutes natural,
then quick

Total time: 3 hours
15 minutes

PER SERVING:
Calories: 465; Fat: 33g;
Carbohydrates: 11g; Fiber: 3g;
Sugar: 5g; Protein: 27g;
Sodium: 360mg

Brisket is a cut of beef that is found just below the shoulder, making it more muscular and a tougher cut. Pressure cooking with moist heat transforms the brisket into a tender, juicy cut of meat. When cooked, the brisket can be cut into uniform pieces or pulled apart in a more shredded fashion.
Any way you slice it, the result will be amazingly delicious!

6 garlic cloves, minced
1 teaspoon dried oregano
1 teaspoon kosher salt
½ teaspoon red pepper flakes
½ teaspoon freshly ground black pepper
1 (2- to 3-pound) beef brisket
1 tablespoon grapeseed oil
3 carrots, cut into ½-inch pieces
2 parsnips, cut into ½-inch pieces
1 onion, julienned
2 celery stalks, cut into ½-inch pieces
¼ cup red wine vinegar
1 (14½-ounce) can low-sodium diced tomatoes
1½ cups gluten-free beef broth
1 strip orange zest
1 cinnamon stick
½ cup chopped fresh parsley, for garnish

1. In a small bowl, mix together the garlic, oregano, salt, red pepper flakes, and pepper.

2. Season the brisket all over with the mixture. Let sit at room temperature for 1 hour.

3. Press the sauté button on the Instant Pot, allow it to heat up, then pour in the oil.

4. Add the brisket and cook for about 5 minutes on one side, or until browned. Remove the brisket and set aside.

5. Add the carrots, parsnips, onion, and celery. Sauté for 3 minutes, or until softened.

6. Add the vinegar and deglaze: Mix well and scrape up any brown bits on the bottom of the pot.

7. Add the tomatoes with their juices, broth, zest, and cinnamon. Mix well.

8. Nestle the brisket into the mixture. Press the cancel button to stop cooking.

9. Secure the lid and cook on high pressure for 1 hour 15 minutes.

10. After cooking, let the pressure release naturally for 30 minutes, then quick release the remaining pressure. Unlock and remove the lid.

11. Transfer the brisket to a cutting board.

12. Press the sauté button, and simmer the sauce for at least 10 minutes, or until reduced to your desired consistency. Press the cancel button to stop cooking.

13. Slice the brisket and serve with the sauce and vegetables. Garnish with the parsley.

SIMPLE SWAP: A variety of root vegetables work well in this dish. Feel free to swap out the carrots and parsnips for turnips and sweet potatoes.

MOROCCAN LAMB

**DAIRY-FREE,
GLUTEN-FREE**

Serves 4
Prep time: 15 minutes
Pressure cook:
45 minutes high
pressure
Pressure release:
20 minutes natural,
then quick
Total time: 1 hour
40 minutes

PER SERVING: Calories: 385;
Fat: 9g; Carbohydrates: 45g;
Fiber: 9g; Sugar: 20g;
Protein: 32g; Sodium: 550mg

---

2 tablespoons ras el
   hanout, divided
¾ teaspoon kosher salt
1 pound lamb shanks
1 tablespoon
   extra-virgin olive oil
1 onion, julienned
5 garlic cloves, minced
1½ cups gluten-free
   beef broth
2 cups Chickpeas
   (page 135) or canned
   chickpeas
½ cup chopped dried
   apricots
½ cup chopped fresh
   cilantro, for garnish
½ cup pomegranate
   seeds, for garnish

Ras el hanout is a Moroccan spice blend whose name translates to "head of the shop." This aromatic, flavorful spice blend typically contains cinnamon, cumin, coriander, allspice, black pepper, ginger, and salt. Look for it in the spice aisle of your grocery store or find it online. It pairs beautifully with the lamb, and the apricots and pomegranate provide a bright, sweet pop of flavor to round out the dish.

---

1. In a small bowl, mix together 1 tablespoon of ras el hanout and the salt.

2. Season the lamb shanks all over with the mixture.

3. Press the sauté button on the Instant Pot, allow it to heat up, then pour in the oil.

4. Add the onion and sauté for 3 minutes, or until softened.

5. Add the garlic and remaining 1 tablespoon of ras el hanout. Sauté for 30 seconds, or until fragrant.

6. Add the broth and deglaze: Mix well and scrape up any brown bits on the bottom of the pot.

7. Nestle the lamb shanks into the mixture. Press the cancel button to stop cooking.

8. Secure the lid and cook on high pressure for 45 minutes.

9. After cooking, let the pressure release naturally for 20 minutes, then quick release the remaining pressure. Unlock and remove the lid.

10. Transfer the lamb to a cutting board. Remove the meat from the bone, reserving the bone (see tip).

11. Stir in the chickpeas and dried apricots. Press the sauté button and simmer the sauce for about 5 minutes, or until thickened.

12. Add the lamb meat to the Instant Pot. Press the cancel button to stop cooking.

13. Serve the lamb garnished with the cilantro and pomegranate seeds.

SAVE FOR LATER: Once you are done eating, save the lamb shank bones and make lamb stock. Just look at the recipe for Chicken Stock (page 141) and swap out the chicken bones for lamb bones.

WHOLE CHICKEN

**DAIRY-FREE,
GLUTEN-FREE**

Serves 6
Prep time: 5 minutes
Pressure cook:
30 minutes high
pressure
Pressure release:
15 minutes natural,
then quick
Total time: 1 hour
20 minutes

PER SERVING:
Calories: 255; Fat: 25g;
Carbohydrates: 1g; Fiber:
0g; Sugar: 0g; Protein: 29g;
Sodium: 480mg

1 (3- to 4-pound)
   whole chicken, giblets
   removed
2 teaspoons kosher
   salt
1 teaspoon freshly
   ground black pepper
1 tablespoon
   extra-virgin olive oil
½ cup water
6 garlic cloves, peeled
1 bunch rosemary,
   thyme, or sage

There's something cozy about a juicy, tender whole chicken. Sautéing helps lock in the flavor and gives it a golden brown hue, making it look even more appetizing. Serve with Potatoes with Greens (page 40) or Farro with Herby Yogurt (page 48).

1. Season the chicken with the salt and pepper.

2. Press the sauté button on the Instant Pot, allow it to heat up, then pour in the oil.

3. Add the chicken, breast-side down, and cook for 5 minutes. Do not move the chicken!

4. Using tongs or 2 large spoons, carefully turn it over and cook for another 5 minutes, or until browned. Press the cancel button to stop cooking.

5. Add the water, carefully drop in the garlic, and lay the rosemary around and across the top of the chicken.

6. Secure the lid and cook on high pressure for 30 minutes.

7. After cooking, let the pressure release naturally for 15 minutes, then quick release the remaining pressure. Unlock and remove the lid.

8. Transfer the chicken to a large cutting board. Let rest for another 10 minutes, then cut and serve.

SAVE FOR LATER: Add leftover chicken to soup, stew, salads, and more; it keeps in the refrigerator for 5 days. Once all the meat has been cut off, put the carcass in a resealable freezer bag and freeze for up to 3 months. Once you are ready, use the leftover chicken bones to make Chicken Stock (page 141).

GREEN CHICKEN SOUP

**DAIRY-FREE,
GLUTEN-FREE**

Serves 6
Prep time: 20 minutes
Pressure cook:
20 minutes high
pressure
Pressure release:
20 minutes natural,
then quick
Total time: 1 hour
10 minutes

2 pounds bone-in
chicken thighs, skin
removed
4 cups Chicken
Stock (page 141)
or store-bought
gluten-free chicken
stock
1 pound asparagus,
woody ends trimmed,
cut into ½-inch pieces
10 ounces frozen peas
1 onion, diced
2 celery stalks, diced
1 teaspoon dried
thyme
¾ teaspoon kosher salt
¼ teaspoon freshly
ground black pepper
1 bay leaf
1 bunch Swiss chard,
stemmed and
chopped
Crusty bread, for
serving (optional)

Chicken soup gets an upgrade with the addition of some delicious, nutritious, and beautiful green vegetables. This dish is perfect for spring, when all the fresh green produce appears at the farmers' market. To make it heartier, mix in some Basic Brown Rice (page 134) or Basic Beans (page 135).

1. In the Instant Pot, combine the chicken, stock, asparagus, peas, onion, celery, thyme, salt, pepper, and bay leaf. Mix well. Secure the lid and cook on high pressure for 20 minutes.

2. After cooking, let the pressure release naturally for 20 minutes, then quick release the remaining pressure. Unlock and remove the lid.

3. Transfer the chicken to a cutting board. Take the meat off the bone, and return the meat to the pot.

4. Add the Swiss chard and mix well.

5. Ladle the soup into bowls. Serve with crusty bread, if desired.

PER SERVING: Calories: 250; Fat: 7g; Carbohydrates: 11g; Fiber: 3g; Sugar: 5g; Protein: 34g; Sodium: 780mg

SIMPLE SWAP: If fresh peas are available, they make a great addition in place of the frozen peas.

LEMON CHICKEN WITH ROSEMARY

DAIRY-FREE, GLUTEN-FREE

Serves 4
Prep time: 10 minutes
Pressure cook:
15 minutes high pressure
Pressure release: Quick
Total time: 40 to 45 minutes

4 boneless, skinless chicken thighs (1 to 1½ pounds)
1 tablespoon chopped fresh rosemary leaves
1 tablespoon chopped fresh thyme leaves
1 teaspoon kosher salt
¼ teaspoon freshly ground black pepper
1 tablespoon extra-virgin olive oil
½ cup white wine
½ cup Chicken Stock (page 141) or store-bought gluten-free chicken stock
¼ cup freshly squeezed lemon juice

Lemon and rosemary are a winning combination in this recipe. Serve this dish with Basic Brown Rice (page 134) to soak up the sauce, or pair it with Bean Salad (page 44) and some pita bread for a light lunch or dinner.

1. Season the chicken with the rosemary, thyme, salt, and pepper.

2. Press the sauté button on the Instant Pot, allow it to heat up, then pour in the oil.

3. Add the chicken and cook for about 3 minutes per side, or until browned on both sides.

4. Add the wine, stock, and lemon juice. Press the cancel button to stop cooking.

5. Secure the lid and cook on high pressure for 15 minutes.

6. After cooking, quick release the pressure. Unlock and remove the lid.

7. Using 2 forks, shred the chicken. Serve immediately.

PER SERVING: Calories: 260; Fat: 10g; Carbohydrates: 2g; Fiber: 0g; Sugar: 1g; Protein: 34g; Sodium: 515mg

SAVE FOR LATER: Leftovers can be stored in an air-tight container for up to 5 days in the refrigerator or up to 3 months in the freezer.

SIMPLE SWAP: Boneless, skinless chicken breasts can be used in place of the chicken thighs.

DECONSTRUCTED LAMB-STUFFED CABBAGE

DAIRY-FREE, GLUTEN-FREE

Serves 4

Prep time: 20 minutes

Pressure cook: 20 minutes high pressure

Pressure release: 10 minutes natural, then quick

Total time: 1 hour 10 minutes

PER SERVING: Calories: 340; Fat: 13g; Carbohydrates: 31g; Fiber: 8g; Sugar: 12g; Protein: 24g; Sodium: 480mg

1 tablespoon extra-virgin olive oil

1 pound ground lamb

1 teaspoon kosher salt

¼ teaspoon freshly ground black pepper

1 onion, diced

4 garlic cloves, minced

1 teaspoon sumac

½ teaspoon ground cinnamon

1 head green cabbage, cored and chopped

¾ cup brown rice

½ cup gluten-free beef stock

Juice of 1 lemon

Stuffed cabbage rolls, also known as malfouf, are a traditional Lebanese dish. I've deconstructed them to create a variation that works well in the Instant Pot. Pair this recipe with some roasted sweet potatoes to round out the meal.

1. Press the sauté button on the Instant Pot, allow it to heat up, then pour in the oil.

2. Add the lamb. Season with the salt and pepper. Cook for about 5 minutes, or until browned.

3. Add the onion and sauté for 3 minutes, or until softened.

4. Add the garlic, sumac, and cinnamon. Sauté for 30 seconds, or until fragrant.

5. Add the cabbage, rice, and stock. Press the cancel button to stop cooking.

6. Secure the lid and cook on high pressure for 20 minutes.

7. After cooking, let the pressure release naturally for 10 minutes, then quick release the remaining pressure. Unlock and remove the lid.

8. Add the lemon juice, mix well, then serve.

SIMPLE SWAP: Any ground meat or poultry works well in this recipe.

LAMB MEAT LOAF WITH TAHINI SAUCE

Serves 4
Prep time: 15 minutes
Pressure cook:
25 minutes high
pressure
Pressure release:
20 minutes natural,
then quick
Total time: 1 hour
20 minutes

PER SERVING: Calories: 535;
Fat: 38g; Carbohydrates: 19g;
Fiber: 3g; Sugar: 5g;
Protein: 28g; Sodium: 435mg

A mini loaf pan fits this lamb meat loaf perfectly in an Instant Pot. If you don't have a mini loaf pan, a 7-inch round cake pan works well. Pair this scrumptious recipe with Potatoes with Greens (page 40) for a well-balanced Mediterranean meal.

Olive oil cooking spray, for coating the loaf pan
1 pound ground lamb
⅓ cup bread crumbs
¼ cup Vegetable Stock (page 140) or store-bought vegetable stock
¼ cup minced onion
¼ cup minced fresh mint leaves
1 large egg, beaten
1 garlic clove, minced
2 teaspoons ground cumin
1 teaspoon ground coriander
1 teaspoon kosher salt, divided
½ teaspoon freshly ground black pepper
½ teaspoon ground cinnamon
1½ cups water
½ cup Plain Yogurt (page 137) or store-bought plain yogurt
⅓ cup tahini
¼ cup freshly squeezed lemon juice

1. Spray a mini loaf pan with cooking spray.

2. In a medium bowl, mix together the lamb, bread crumbs, stock, onion, mint, egg, garlic, cumin, coriander, ½ teaspoon of salt, the pepper, and cinnamon.

3. Pack the mixture into the prepared loaf pan, and cover tightly with aluminum foil.

4. Pour the water into the Instant Pot, place the steam trivet inside, and place the loaf pan on top of the trivet. Secure the lid and cook on high pressure for 25 minutes.

5. After cooking, let the pressure release naturally for 20 minutes, then quick release the remaining pressure. Unlock and remove the lid. Remove the loaf pan, uncover, and let cool for 10 minutes.

6. While the lamb is cooking, make the tahini sauce: In a small bowl, mix together the yogurt, tahini, lemon juice, and remaining ½ teaspoon of salt.

7. Pour the tahini sauce over the meat loaf, or serve on the side.

TROUBLESHOOTING TIP: To ensure lamb is cooked through properly, use an instant-read thermometer. It should register at least 160°F.

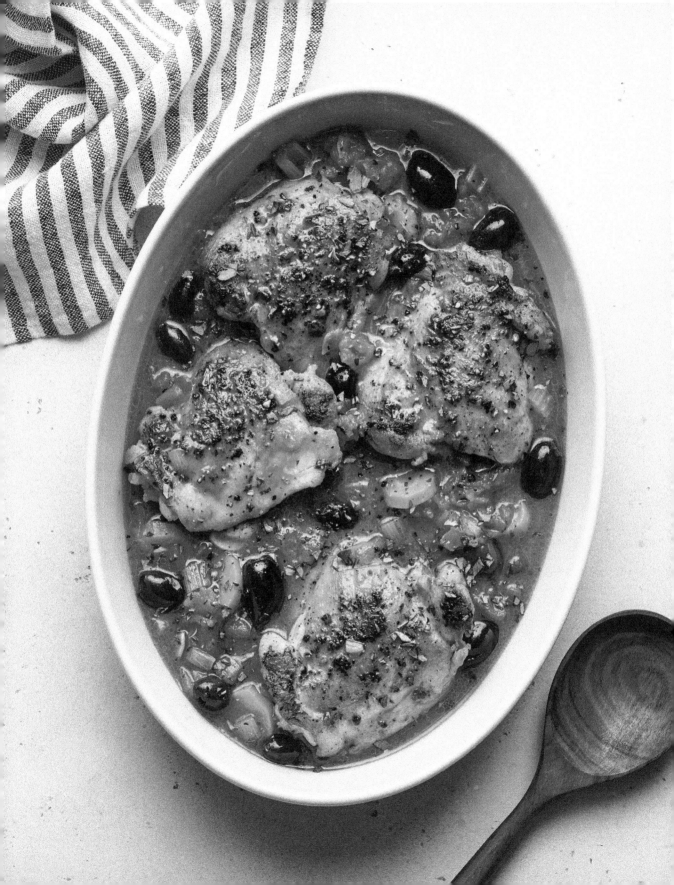

BRAISED CHICKEN WITH TOMATO AND OLIVES

**DAIRY-FREE,
GLUTEN-FREE**

Serves 4
Prep time: 15 minutes
Pressure cook:
20 minutes high
pressure
**Pressure
release:** Quick
Total time: 55 minutes
to 1 hour

PER SERVING: Calories: 450;
Fat: 20g; Carbohydrates: 15g;
Fiber: 3g; Sugar: 8g;
Protein: 47g; Sodium: 900mg

Olives, known as a rich source of healthy fats, are a staple in the Mediterranean diet. They are often cured or pickled by being immersed in water, oil, or brine. Olive oil is made by crushing and pressing olives. Both olives and olive oil are excellent sources of healthy monounsaturated fatty acids, vitamin E, and flavonoids. Garnish the finished dish with parsley, if desired.

4 bone-in chicken thighs, skin removed (2 to
  2½ pounds)
1 teaspoon kosher salt
¼ teaspoon freshly ground black pepper
2 tablespoons extra-virgin olive oil, divided
1 onion, diced
1 celery stalk, diced
1 carrot, diced
2 garlic cloves, minced
½ cup white wine
1 (28-ounce) can low-sodium whole tomatoes
¾ cup chopped pitted black olives
¼ cup Chicken Stock (page 141) or store-bought
  gluten-free chicken stock
2 teaspoons dried basil
2 teaspoons dried oregano
⅛ teaspoon red pepper flakes

1. Season the chicken with the salt and pepper.

2. Press the sauté button on the Instant Pot, allow it to heat up, then pour in 1 tablespoon of oil.

3. Add the chicken and cook on one side for about 5 minutes, or until browned. Remove the chicken and set aside.

continued ➤

4. Heat the remaining 1 tablespoon of oil.

5. Add the onion, celery, and carrot. Sauté for 5 minutes, or until softened.

6. Add the garlic and sauté for 30 seconds, or until fragrant.

7. Add the wine and deglaze: Mix well and scrape up any brown bits on the bottom of the pot.

8. Add the tomatoes with their juices, olives, stock, basil, oregano, and red pepper flakes. Mix well.

9. Return the chicken to the pot. Press the cancel button to stop cooking.

10. Secure the lid and cook on high pressure for 20 minutes.

11. After cooking, quick release the pressure. Unlock and remove the lid.

12. Transfer the chicken to a serving dish. (Optional: Press the sauté button and simmer the sauce until the desired consistency is reached.) Serve immediately.

SAVE FOR LATER: Leftovers can be stored in an airtight container for up to 5 days in the refrigerator or up to 3 months in the freezer.

CHICKEN WITH MUSHROOMS

DAIRY-FREE, GLUTEN-FREE

Serves 4
Prep time: 15 minutes
Pressure cook: 15 minutes high pressure
Pressure release: Quick
Total time: 50 to 55 minutes

PER SERVING: Calories: 375; Fat: 13g; Carbohydrates: 9g; Fiber: 1g; Sugar: 4g; Protein: 55g; Sodium: 540mg

4 bone-in chicken breasts, skin removed (2 to 2½ pounds)
1 teaspoon kosher salt
¼ teaspoon freshly ground black pepper
2 tablespoons extra-virgin olive oil, divided
1 pound cremini mushrooms, thinly sliced
1 onion, diced
1 cup Chicken Stock (page 141) or store-bought gluten-free chicken stock
1 tablespoon Italian seasoning

Mushrooms add an earthy flavor to this dish, pair beautifully with chicken, and are an excellent source of many nutrients, including selenium, zinc, B vitamins, and potassium. Serve with lemon wedges and a sprinkle of parsley for an extra pop.

1. Season the chicken with the salt and pepper.

2. Press the sauté button on the Instant Pot, allow it to heat up, then pour in 1 tablespoon of oil.

3. Add the chicken and cook on one side for about 5 minutes, or until browned. Remove the chicken and set aside.

4. Heat the remaining 1 tablespoon of oil.

5. Add the mushrooms and onion. Sauté for 8 to 10 minutes, or until softened.

6. Add the stock and Italian seasoning. Deglaze: Mix well and scrape up any brown bits on the bottom of the pot.

7. Return the chicken to the Instant Pot. Press the cancel button to stop cooking.

8. Secure the lid and cook on high pressure for 15 minutes.

9. After cooking, quick release the pressure. Unlock and remove the lid.

10. Transfer the chicken to a serving dish. (Optional: Press the sauté button and simmer the sauce until your desired consistency is reached.) Serve immediately.

SIMPLE SWAP: Feel free to swap out the chicken breasts for bone-in, skinless chicken thighs and drumsticks.

PORK RAGÙ

**DAIRY-FREE,
GLUTEN-FREE**

Serves 4
Prep time: 15 minutes
Pressure cook:
45 minutes high
pressure
Pressure release:
15 minutes natural,
then quick
Total time: 1 hour
35 minutes

PER SERVING: Calories: 305;
Fat: 11g; Carbohydrates: 19g;
Fiber: 4g; Sugar: 12g;
Protein: 26g; Sodium: 410mg

This version of Pork Ragù uses the leaner tenderloin cut. A pork shoulder can also be used for a richer ragù; just be sure to adjust the amounts of the other ingredients accordingly based on the size of the cut of pork. Serve this dish over pasta, vegetable noodles, or whole grains, like Basic Brown Rice (page 134).

1 pound pork tenderloin
1 teaspoon kosher salt
½ teaspoon freshly ground black pepper
2 tablespoons extra-virgin olive oil, divided
1 onion, diced
5 garlic cloves, minced
½ cup white wine
1 (28-ounce) can low-sodium whole tomatoes
½ cup Vegetable Stock (page 140) or store-bought vegetable stock
1 tablespoon Italian seasoning
½ teaspoon fennel seeds
¼ teaspoon red pepper flakes

1. Season the pork with the salt and pepper.

2. Press the sauté button on the Instant Pot, allow it to heat up, then pour in 1 tablespoon of oil.

3. Add the pork and cook on 2 sides for about 3 minutes per side, or until browned. Remove the pork and set aside.

4. Heat the remaining 1 tablespoon of oil.

5. Add the onion and sauté for 2 minutes, or until softened.

6. Add the garlic and sauté for 30 seconds, or until fragrant.

7. Add the wine and deglaze: Mix well and scrape up any brown bits on the bottom of the pot.

8. Add the tomatoes with their juices, stock, Italian seasoning, fennel seeds, and red pepper flakes. Mix well.

9. Return the pork to the pot. Press the cancel button to stop cooking.

10. Secure the lid and cook on high pressure for 45 minutes.

11. After cooking, let the pressure release naturally for 15 minutes, then quick release the remaining pressure. Unlock and remove the lid.

12. Using 2 forks, shred the pork. Serve immediately.

SAVE FOR LATER: Put leftovers in an airtight container and refrigerate for up to 5 days, or freeze for up to 3 months.

CHICKEN WITH PEPPERS

**DAIRY-FREE,
GLUTEN-FREE**

Serves 4
Prep time: 20 minutes
Pressure cook:
15 minutes high
pressure
**Pressure
release:** Quick
Total time: 55 minutes
to 1 hour

PER SERVING: Calories: 255;
Fat: 12g; Carbohydrates: 9g;
Fiber: 2g; Sugar: 4g;
Protein: 24g; Sodium: 465mg

Bell peppers, available in a range of colors, are widely used throughout the Mediterranean region. Red, orange, and yellow bell peppers are sweeter, whereas green and purple bell peppers have a slightly bitter flavor. Here's a fun fact: Did you know that green bell peppers that are left on the vine to sweeten become red bell peppers? Both paprika and pimento are also prepared from bell peppers.

1 pound boneless, skinless chicken thighs
1 teaspoon kosher salt
¼ teaspoon freshly ground black pepper
2 tablespoons extra-virgin olive oil, divided
1 onion, julienned
1 green bell pepper, julienned
1 red bell pepper, julienned
1 tablespoon fresh oregano leaves or 1 teaspoon
   dried oregano
2 garlic cloves, minced
½ cup red wine
½ cup Chicken Stock (page 141) or store-bought
   gluten-free chicken stock
¼ cup chopped fresh parsley, for garnish

1. Season the chicken with the salt and pepper.

2. Press the sauté button on the Instant Pot, allow it
    to heat up, then pour in 1 tablespoon of oil.

3. Add the chicken and cook for 2 to 3 minutes per
    side, or until browned on both sides. Remove the
    chicken and set aside.

4. Heat the remaining 1 tablespoon of oil.

5. Add the onion, green bell pepper, and red bell pepper. Sauté for 5 minutes, or until softened.

6. Add the oregano and garlic. Sauté for 30 seconds, or until fragrant.

7. Add the wine and deglaze: Mix well and scrape up any brown bits on the bottom of the pot.

8. Add the stock and chicken. Press the cancel button to stop cooking.

9. Secure the lid and cook on high pressure for 15 minutes.

10. After cooking, quick release the pressure. Unlock and remove the lid.

11. Transfer the chicken to a serving dish. (Optional: Press the sauté button and simmer the sauce until the desired consistency is reached.) Garnish with the parsley. Serve immediately.

SIMPLE SWAP: Feel free to use any color of bell peppers you like.

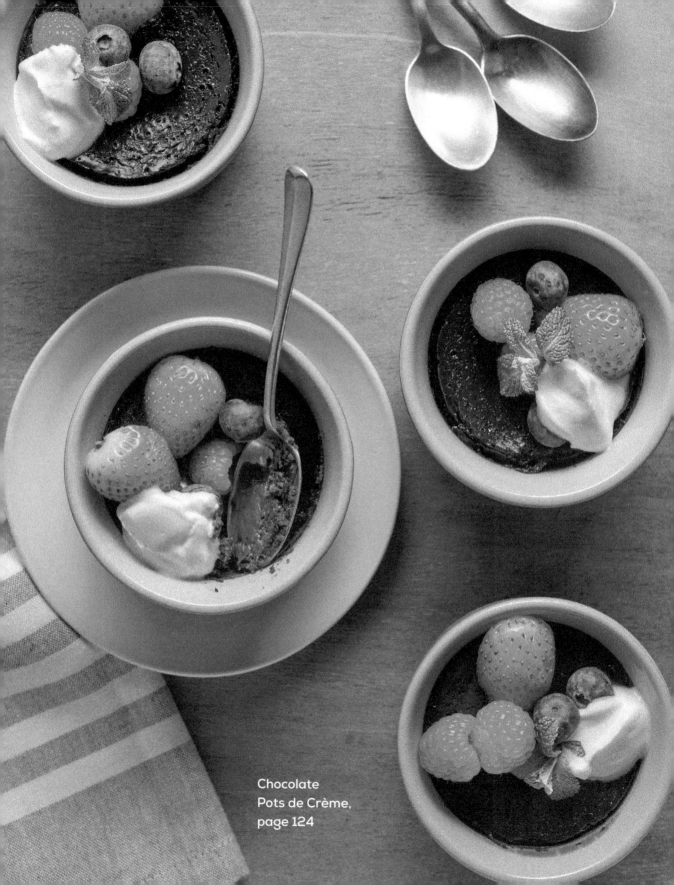

Chocolate
Pots de Crème,
page 124

CHAPTER EIGHT

DESSERT

Baked Apples 120

Berry Compote with Yogurt 121

Poached Pears with Cardamom 122

Chocolate Pots de Crème. 124

Nut and Fig "Pudding" with Yogurt Cream. 126

Custard with Roasted Fruit .128

Rice Pudding. 130

BAKED APPLES

**DAIRY-FREE,
GLUTEN-FREE**

Serves 4
Prep time: 15 minutes
Pressure cook:
10 minutes high
pressure
Pressure release:
15 minutes natural,
then quick
Total time: 50 minutes

PER SERVING: Calories: 180;
Fat: 3g; Carbohydrates: 38g;
Fiber: 6g; Sugar: 28g;
Protein: 2g; Sodium: 5mg

1 cup water
4 Granny Smith apples,
  cored
2 tablespoons raisins
2 tablespoons
  chopped walnuts
4 teaspoons honey
1 teaspoon ground
  cinnamon
Olive oil cooking spray,
  for coating the
  steam rack

Apples hold up well in the Instant Pot and provide a nice sweet treat. Granny Smith apples are tart and keep their texture well during cooking. However, some other varieties, such as Golden Delicious and Fuji, are best eaten raw.

1. Pour the water into the Instant Pot.

2. Fill the apples with the raisins, walnuts, honey, and cinnamon.

3. Coat the steam rack with cooking spray, and put it inside the pot, handles extending up. Place the apples on the prepared steam rack.

4. Secure the lid and cook on high pressure for 10 minutes.

5. After cooking, let the pressure release naturally for 15 minutes, then quick release the remaining pressure. Unlock and remove the lid.

6. Carefully remove the steam rack with the apples and serve warm.

SIMPLE SWAP: Swap out the walnuts and raisins for any nuts and dried fruit you like.

BERRY COMPOTE WITH YOGURT

GLUTEN-FREE
Serves 4
Prep time: 15 minutes
Pressure cook:
2 minutes high
pressure
Pressure release:
15 minutes natural,
then quick
Total time: 40 to
45 minutes

PER SERVING: Calories:
220; Fat: 3g; Carbohydrates:
43g; Fiber: 10g; Sugar: 30g;
Protein: 8g; Sodium: 240mg

2 pounds mixed
   berries
2 tablespoons maple
   syrup
2 tablespoons maple
   sugar
Grated zest of ½ lemon
Juice of ½ lemon
Grated zest of
   ½ orange
Juice of ½ orange
2 cups Plain Yogurt
   (page 137) or
   store-bought plain
   yogurt

This dish is a delicious and nutritious dessert, snack, or breakfast. To bump up the fiber content, add a handful of nuts or seeds. Or add a pop of color and flavor with some chopped mint. Berry compote is a great recipe to batch up and keep on hand in the freezer.

1. In the Instant Pot, combine the berries, maple syrup, maple sugar, lemon zest, lemon juice, orange zest, and orange juice. Mix well.

2. Secure the lid and cook on high pressure for 2 minutes.

3. After cooking, let the pressure release naturally for 15 minutes, then quick release the remaining pressure. Unlock and remove the lid, then mix well.

4. If desired, press the sauté button, and simmer the mixture to thicken. Press the cancel button to stop cooking.

5. Serve the compote with the yogurt.

SAVE FOR LATER: The berry compote can be stored in an airtight container for up to 1 week in the refrigerator or up to 6 months in the freezer.

POACHED PEARS WITH CARDAMOM

**DAIRY-FREE,
GLUTEN-FREE**

Serves 4
Prep time: 10 minutes
Pressure cook:
8 minutes high
pressure
**Pressure
release:** Quick
Total time: 45 minutes

4 firm pears, peeled
2 cups water
2 cups dry white wine
½ cup granulated
  sugar
2 tablespoons freshly
  squeezed lemon juice
10 cardamom pods,
  lightly crushed, or
  1 teaspoon ground
  cardamom
Pinch saffron threads
⅛ teaspoon kosher salt
½ cup pistachios,
  chopped

SIMPLE SWAP: If you
don't have pistachios,
use any nuts or seeds
you like. You can also top
the pears with a dollop
of yogurt, crème fraîche,
or whipped cream in
addition to or in place of
the nuts.

Poached pears are one of my favorite fruit-based desserts. My version uses white wine and cardamom, adding spicy, herbal, fragrant notes to the dish. If you do not have cardamom, try a 1-inch knob of peeled ginger and a cinnamon stick instead. Red wine may also be used in place of the white wine if preferred.

1. Using a melon baller or spoon, scoop out the seeds and core from the bottom of each pear.

2. In the Instant Pot, combine the water, wine, sugar, lemon juice, cardamom, saffron, and salt. Mix well. Press the sauté button, and bring to a simmer.

3. Add the pears and press the cancel button to stop cooking.

4. Secure the lid and cook on high pressure for 8 minutes.

5. After cooking, quick release the pressure. Unlock and remove the lid.

6. Transfer the pears to serving dishes.

7. Press the sauté button and bring the liquid to a boil. Reduce by about half. Press the cancel button to stop cooking.

8. While the liquid boils, in a small skillet, toast the pistachios over medium heat for about 5 minutes, or until golden brown. Remove from the heat.

9. Ladle the sauce over each pear and garnish with the pistachios.

PER SERVING: Calories: 260; Fat: 7g; Carbohydrates: 43g; Fiber: 6g; Sugar: 35g; Protein: 4g; Sodium: 38mg

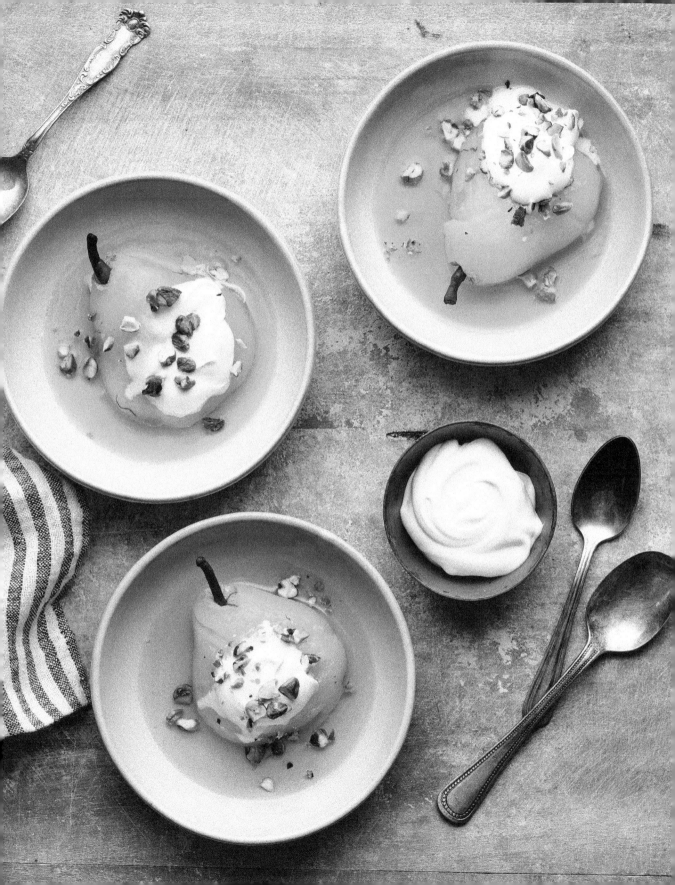

CHOCOLATE POTS DE CRÈME

GLUTEN-FREE
Serves 4
Prep time: 15 minutes
Pressure cook:
8 minutes high
pressure
Pressure release:
20 minutes natural,
then quick
Total time: 1 hour
55 minutes

PER SERVING: Calories: 475;
Fat: 44g; Carbohydrates: 16g;
Fiber: 2g; Sugar: 12g;
Protein: 6g; Sodium: 115mg

These sweet treats are sure to be a crowd-pleaser. Serve them with berries and a dollop of crème fraîche or Plain Yogurt (page 137) and some fresh mint. I like using maple sugar because it adds a nice flavor to the dish, but feel free to swap it out for brown sugar or coconut sugar.

1½ cups heavy cream, divided
2 ounces dark chocolate (70 percent), chopped
Pinch cayenne pepper
4 large egg yolks
3 tablespoons maple sugar
1 teaspoon vanilla extract
¼ teaspoon kosher salt
1½ cups water

1. In a small saucepan, combine ¼ cup of heavy cream and the chocolate. Melt together over low heat, whisking occasionally. Remove from the heat.

2. Whisk in the remaining 1¼ cups of heavy cream and the cayenne.

3. In a medium bowl, whisk together the egg yolks, maple sugar, vanilla, and salt.

4. Whisking continuously, slowly add some of the chocolate-cream mixture until everything is combined. Pour into 4 ramekins, and cover each tightly with aluminum foil.

5. Pour the water into the Instant Pot. Put a steam rack inside the pot, handles extending up. Place the ramekins on the steam rack.

6. Secure the lid and cook on high pressure for 8 minutes.

7. After cooking, let the pressure release naturally for 20 minutes, then quick release the remaining pressure. Unlock and remove the lid.

8. Carefully remove the ramekins, remove the foil, and cool before serving.

SIMPLE SWAP: If you prefer milk chocolate or white chocolate, feel free to swap out the dark chocolate.

NUT AND FIG "PUDDING" WITH YOGURT CREAM

GLUTEN-FREE
Serves 6
Prep time: 15 minutes
Pressure cook:
5 minutes high
pressure
**Pressure
release:** Quick
Total time: 40 to
45 minutes

PER SERVING: Calories: 370;
Fat: 31g; Carbohydrates: 22g;
Fiber: 5g; Sugar: 15g;
Protein: 6g; Sodium: 65mg

Fig trees are native to the Mediterranean region and are also the world's first cultivated tree. Figs vary in color and texture depending on the variety, ranging from light green to purple or yellow skin and pink to amber or red flesh. Some of the most popular fig types are Black Mission, Calimyrna, Brown Turkey, and Adriatic.

FOR THE PUDDING
1 pound figs, stemmed and chopped
1 cup water
½ cup chopped walnuts
½ cup chopped pistachios
½ cup chopped pecans
¼ cup ground espresso (optional)
3 tablespoons unsalted butter, melted
½ teaspoon ground cardamom
¼ teaspoon ground ginger
¼ teaspoon ground cinnamon
¼ teaspoon kosher salt

FOR THE YOGURT CREAM
½ cup heavy cream
¼ cup Plain Yogurt (page 137) or store-bought
   plain yogurt
1 teaspoon confectioners' sugar

TO MAKE THE PUDDING

1. In the Instant Pot, combine the figs and water. Secure the lid and cook on high pressure for 5 minutes.

2. After cooking, quick release the pressure. Unlock and remove the lid.

3. Mash together the figs and water.

4. Add the walnuts, pistachios, pecans, espresso (if using), butter, cardamom, ginger, cinnamon, and salt. Press the sauté button and simmer, stirring often, for 10 minutes, or until thickened. Press the cancel button to stop cooking.

TO MAKE THE YOGURT CREAM

5. In a medium bowl, combine the heavy cream, yogurt, and sugar. Whisk for about 2 minutes, or until soft peaks form.

6. Divide the pudding among bowls. Top with the yogurt cream.

SIMPLE SWAP:
Feel free to swap out any of the nuts and use whatever nuts and seeds you like.

CUSTARD WITH ROASTED FRUIT

GLUTEN-FREE

Serves 4

Prep time: 15 minutes

Pressure cook:
6 minutes high
pressure

Pressure release:
20 minutes natural,
then quick

Total time: 1 hour
30 minutes

PER SERVING: Calories: 160;
Fat: 5g; Carbohydrates: 22g;
Fiber: 2g; Sugar: 20g;
Protein: 7g; Sodium: 250mg

Roasted fruit is amazingly delicious on its own, but it pairs beautifully with this custard. You can make the custard the day before and serve it chilled with warm roasted fruit. Basil also goes nicely with this dessert in place of the mint.

FOR THE CUSTARD

1¾ cups whole milk

4 large eggs

3 tablespoons granulated sugar

1 teaspoon vanilla extract

¼ teaspoon kosher salt

1½ cups water

FOR THE ROASTED FRUIT

1 tablespoon maple syrup

1 teaspoon extra-virgin olive oil

¼ teaspoon kosher salt

½ cup strawberries, stemmed

½ cup raspberries

¼ cup chopped fresh mint leaves, for garnish

TO MAKE THE CUSTARD

1. In a medium bowl, whisk together the milk, eggs, sugar, vanilla, and salt. Pour into 4 ramekins, and cover tightly with aluminum foil.

2. Pour the water into the Instant Pot. Put a steam rack inside the pot, handles extending up. Place the ramekins on the steam rack.

3. Secure the lid and cook on high pressure for 6 minutes.

4. After cooking, let the pressure release naturally for 20 minutes, then quick release the remaining pressure. Unlock and remove the lid.

5. Carefully remove the ramekins, remove the foil, and let cool.

TO MAKE THE ROASTED FRUIT

6. While the custard is cooking, preheat the oven to 250°F. Line a baking sheet with parchment paper or foil.

7. In a large bowl, whisk together the maple syrup, oil, and salt.

8. Add the berries and carefully toss together.

9. Spread the berries out in a single layer on the prepared baking sheet.

10. Transfer the baking sheet to the oven and roast for 1 hour 30 minutes, or until the fruit is reduced and soft. Remove from the oven.

11. Serve the custard with the roasted fruit, and garnish with the mint.

SIMPLE SWAP: For a delicious twist, swap out the vanilla extract for almond extract.

RICE PUDDING

GLUTEN-FREE
Serves 4
Prep time: 15 minutes
Pressure cook:
10 minutes high
pressure
Pressure release:
15 minutes natural,
then quick
Total time: 1 hour
5 minutes

PER SERVING: Calories: 355;
Fat: 13g; Carbohydrates: 48g;
Fiber: 1g; Sugar: 19g;
Protein: 12g; Sodium: 200mg

1 tablespoon unsalted
    butter
⅔ cup Arborio rice
1 (12-ounce) can
    evaporated reduced
    fat milk
½ cup water
⅓ cup maple sugar
1 cinnamon stick
1 tablespoon
    granulated sugar
1 teaspoon vanilla
    extract
¼ teaspoon kosher salt
¼ cup heavy cream
1 large egg
1 large egg yolk

Rice pudding can be found throughout the Mediterranean, with slight variations depending on the region. Some areas use nutmeg or cardamom and others use orange blossom water or rose water. Regardless of where you are, the basics of rice pudding remain the same.

1. Press the sauté button on the Instant Pot, allow it to heat up, then drop in the butter.

2. Once the butter has melted, add the rice, and sauté for 1 minute.

3. Add the evaporated milk, water, maple sugar, cinnamon, sugar, vanilla, and salt. Mix well. Press the cancel button to stop cooking.

4. Secure the lid and cook on high pressure for 10 minutes.

5. After cooking, let the pressure release naturally for 15 minutes, then quick release the remaining pressure. Unlock and remove the lid, then mix well. Remove the cinnamon stick.

6. In a small bowl, whisk together the heavy cream, egg, and egg yolk.

7. Add ½ cup of the rice mixture to the egg mixture, and mix.

8. Add the egg and rice mixture to the rest of the rice and mix together well. Let sit for 5 to 10 minutes.

9. Serve warm, or transfer to airtight containers and chill in the refrigerator before serving.

TROUBLESHOOTING TIP: Add the hot rice mixture carefully to the egg mixture, being sure to temper properly and not scramble the egg. This can be done by adding a small amount at a time and mixing well before adding more.

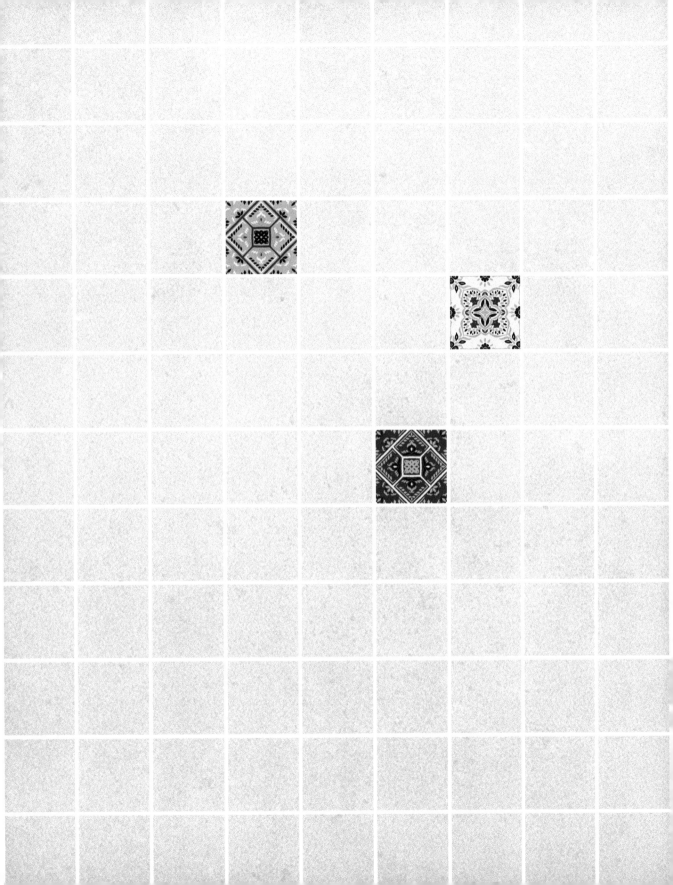

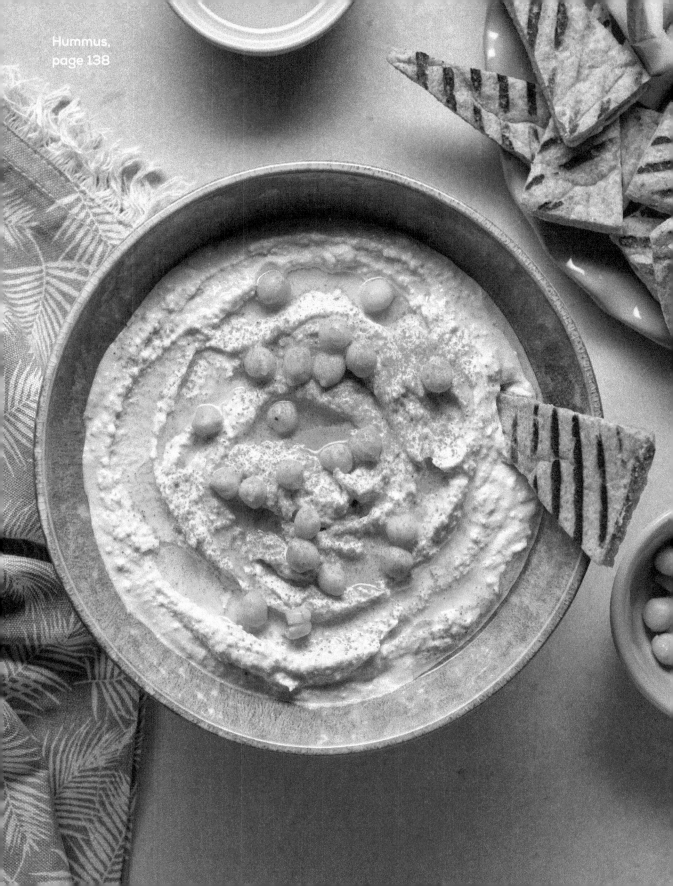

Hummus,
page 138

CHAPTER NINE

SAUCES AND STAPLES

Basic Brown Rice 134

Basic Beans 135

Hard- and Soft-Boiled Eggs 136

Plain Yogurt 137

Hummus 138

Tzatziki 139

Vegetable Stock. 140

Chicken Stock 141

Basil-Walnut Pesto 142

Tahini Dressing. 144

BASIC BROWN RICE

**DAIRY-FREE,
GLUTEN-FREE**

Makes 3 cups

Prep time: 5 minutes

Pressure cook:
15 minutes low
pressure

Pressure release:
20 minutes natural,
then quick

Total time: 45 to
50 minutes

PER SERVING (½ CUP):
Calories: 190; Fat: 4g;
Carbohydrates: 37g;
Fiber: 3g; Sugar: 0g;
Protein: 3g; Sodium: 200mg

---

1 tablespoon
extra-virgin olive oil

1½ cups long-grain
brown rice, rinsed

1 teaspoon kosher salt

6 cups water

Brown rice is a wonderfully versatile grain able to complement practically any food. There are many different varieties of rice, but brown rice is one of the most nutritious. It is chock-full of B vitamins, manganese, selenium, iron, dietary fiber, and protein in addition to many other nutrients.

1. Press the sauté button on the Instant Pot, allow it to heat up, then pour in the oil.

2. Add the rice and salt. Sauté for 30 seconds.

3. Add the water, and mix well. Press the cancel button to stop cooking.

4. Secure the lid and cook on low pressure for 15 minutes.

5. After cooking, let the pressure release naturally for 20 minutes, then quick release any remaining pressure. Unlock and remove the lid.

6. Mix well and taste for doneness. If there is liquid remaining in the pot, drain it through a fine-mesh strainer.

SAVE FOR LATER: To save rice, first spread it on a rimmed baking sheet to cool to room temperature quickly. Store it in airtight containers or resealable freezer bags, label with the name and date, and put in the refrigerator for up to 1 week or in the freezer for up to 3 months.

BASIC BEANS

**DAIRY-FREE,
GLUTEN-FREE**

Makes 6 cups
Prep time: 5 minutes
Pressure cook:
30 minutes high
pressure
Pressure release:
30 minutes natural,
then quick
Total time: 1 hour
15 minutes

PER SERVING (½ CUP):
Calories: 125; Fat: 0g;
Carbohydrates: 23g;
Fiber: 9g; Sugar: 1g;
Protein: 9g; Sodium: 60mg

6 cups water
**1 pound dried beans
   of choice, picked
   through and rinsed**
½ teaspoon kosher salt

Beans are a staple throughout the Mediterranean region and are an excellent source of plant-based protein. Most dried beans, including chickpeas, cannellini beans, and kidney beans, should take 30 minutes to cook; however, if you open the lid and find your beans still a bit too hard for your liking, simply turn on the sauté function and simmer for 5 to 10 minutes.

1. In the Instant Pot, combine the water, beans, and salt. Secure the lid and cook on high pressure for 30 minutes.

2. After cooking, let the pressure release naturally for 30 minutes, then quick release the remaining pressure. Unlock and remove the lid, then mix well.

SAVE FOR LATER: Store beans in airtight containers, with or without liquid, for up to 1 week in the refrigerator or up to 6 months in the freezer.

HARD- AND SOFT-BOILED EGGS

DAIRY-FREE, GLUTEN-FREE

Serves 6

Prep time: 5 minutes

Pressure cook: 3 to 7 minutes high pressure

Pressure release: Quick

Total time: 15 to 25 minutes

PER SERVING (1 EGG):
Calories: 70; Fat: 5g;
Carbohydrates: 0g; Fiber: 0g;
Sugar: 0g; Protein: 6g;
Sodium: 70mg

---

6 large eggs

Eggs are an excellent source of protein, clocking in at 6 grams per large egg. They also have many essential vitamins and minerals, including vitamin B_{12}, choline, selenium, and biotin. Making a dozen hard-boiled eggs in the Instant Pot is a breeze. Keep them in the refrigerator to add to meals and snacks all week.

---

1. Fill a large bowl with ice water.

2. Pour 1 cup of water into the Instant Pot. Put a steam rack in the pot, and place the eggs carefully on top. Secure the lid and cook on high pressure for 3 minutes (soft-boiled), 4 to 5 minutes (medium-boiled), or 6 to 7 minutes (hard-boiled).

3. After cooking, quick release the pressure. Unlock and remove the lid.

4. Transfer the eggs immediately to the ice water bath for 1 to 2 minutes.

SAVE FOR LATER: If not eating right away, leave in the shell and refrigerate for up to 5 days.

PLAIN YOGURT

GLUTEN-FREE
Makes 5 cups
Prep time: 10 minutes
Pressure cook: 8 hours
30 minutes yogurt
pressure setting
Total time: 9 hours,
plus at least 8 hours
to chill

PER SERVING (½ CUP):
Calories: 65; Fat: 2g;
Carbohydrates: 6g; Fiber: 0g;
Sugar: 6g; Protein: 4g;
Sodium: 60mg

---

5 cups reduced-fat or
whole milk
2 tablespoons plain
yogurt with live
cultures

Yogurt is a staple in the Mediterranean diet and, like other dairy products, is a very good source of protein, calcium, phosphorous, vitamin B$_{12}$, and many other nutrients. Yogurt is a fermented dairy product, meaning it is made by adding bacterial cultures to milk that convert the lactose into lactic acid. This process creates yogurt's tart and sour flavor and unique texture. As you'll see from the recipe, the process takes some time but is very easy to do—and it is well worth the wait!

1. Pour the milk into the Instant Pot. Secure the lid, press the yogurt button, and adjust the pressure to boil. This part takes about 30 minutes.

2. Once done, fill a large bowl with ice water. Remove the entire pot, and place it in the ice water bath for 15 minutes, or until the milk chills to 100°F to 115°F.

3. Add the yogurt to the milk and whisk.

4. Remove the pot from the ice bath, dry it off, and place back in the Instant Pot.

5. Press the yogurt button, and set the timer to 8 hours.

6. After cooking, transfer the yogurt to airtight containers and refrigerate for 8 to 10 hours before eating.

SAVE FOR LATER: Yogurt can be stored in airtight containers in the refrigerator for up to 10 days or in the freezer for up to 1 month.

HUMMUS

**DAIRY-FREE,
GLUTEN-FREE**

Makes about 2 cups
Prep time: 15 minutes
Total time: 15 minutes

PER SERVING (¼ CUP):
Calories: 170; Fat: 11g;
Carbohydrates: 14g;
Fiber: 4g; Sugar: 2g;
Protein: 5g; Sodium: 150mg

2 cups Chickpeas
(page 135) or canned
chickpeas
⅓ cup tahini
Juice of 1 lemon
1 garlic clove, smashed
and peeled
1 teaspoon kosher salt
½ teaspoon ground
cumin
¼ teaspoon freshly
ground black pepper
3 tablespoons
extra-virgin olive oil

Hummus is a staple throughout the Mediterranean region. There are many different variations, such as adding spices like za'atar and sumac or incorporating ingredients like roasted red peppers. Drizzle some nice olive oil on top, sprinkle with your favorite spices, and serve with pita bread and crudités.

1. In a food processor, combine the chickpeas, tahini, lemon juice, garlic, salt, cumin, and pepper. Pulse 8 to 10 times.

2. Continue to process while adding the oil until your desired consistency is reached.

SIMPLE SWAP: Traditional hummus uses chickpeas, but other beans also taste great and work well in this recipe.

TZATZIKI

GLUTEN-FREE
Makes 1½ cups
Prep time: 15 minutes
Total time: 15 minutes

PER SERVING (¼ CUP):
Calories: 55; Fat: 3g;
Carbohydrates: 5g; Fiber: 0g;
Sugar: 4g; Protein: 2g;
Sodium: 175mg

SAVE FOR LATER:
Tzatziki should stay fresh
in the refrigerator for up
to 5 days. Just give it a
good stir before serving.

I love the refreshing mix of cucumbers, yogurt, and
herbs. And the zingy lemon makes the whole dish
pop! Here's a tip: Grate the cucumber using the
large holes of a box grater for a chunkier version
or the small holes for a smoother version. Pair this
with pita bread, vegetables, or roasted meat or
poultry.

2 Persian cucumbers, grated
1 cup Plain Yogurt (page 137) or store-bought
   plain yogurt
2 tablespoons chopped fresh dill
2 tablespoons chopped fresh mint leaves
Juice of ½ lemon
1 tablespoon extra-virgin olive oil
1 garlic clove, grated
¾ teaspoon kosher salt

In a medium bowl, combine the cucumbers, yogurt,
dill, mint, lemon juice, oil, garlic, and salt. Mix
together well.

VEGETABLE STOCK

DAIRY-FREE, GLUTEN-FREE

Makes 10 cups
Prep time: 15 minutes
Pressure cook: 1 hour high pressure
Pressure release: 30 minutes natural, then quick
Total time: 2 hours 25 minutes

PER SERVING (½ CUP): Calories: 0; Fat: 0g; Carbohydrates: 0g; Fiber: 0g; Sugar: 0g; Protein: 0g; Sodium: 90mg

2 onions, quartered
2 carrots, quartered
2 celery stalks, cut into 2-inch pieces
1 bunch parsley
6 thyme sprigs
5 garlic cloves, smashed and peeled
1½ teaspoons kosher salt
1 teaspoon black peppercorns
3 bay leaves
10 cups water

Homemade vegetable stock is amazingly flavorful and easy to make and have on hand. During the week, simply save leftover vegetable scraps, put them in a resealable bag, and freeze. Once you have enough vegetables saved up, you can use them in this recipe.

1. In the Instant Pot, combine the onions, carrots, celery, parsley, thyme, garlic, salt, peppercorns, and bay leaves.

2. Add the water, making sure not to go past the "max fill" line. Secure the lid and cook on high pressure for 1 hour.

3. After cooking, let the pressure release naturally for 30 minutes, then quick release the remaining pressure. Unlock and remove the lid, then mix well.

4. Strain the stock through a fine-mesh strainer or colander into a large bowl. Discard the solids, and let the stock cool for 30 minutes.

SAVE FOR LATER: Portion out vegetable stock into airtight containers, and store in the refrigerator for up to 1 week or in the freezer for up to 6 months. If freezing, you can portion out stock into resealable freezer bags and place several in a stack flat on a baking sheet. Once frozen, remove the baking sheet, and keep the frozen stock stacked in the freezer.

CHICKEN STOCK

DAIRY-FREE, GLUTEN-FREE

Makes 10 cups
Prep time: 15 minutes
Pressure cook: 1 hour high pressure
Pressure release: 30 minutes natural, then quick
Total time: 2 hours 25 minutes

PER SERVING (½ CUP):
Calories: 0; Fat: 0g;
Carbohydrates: 0g; Fiber: 0g;
Sugar: 0g; Protein: 0g;
Sodium: 90mg

---

2 to 2½ pounds
   chicken bones
1 onion, quartered
2 carrots, quartered
2 celery stalks, cut into
   2-inch pieces
3 garlic cloves,
   smashed and peeled
1½ teaspoons kosher
   salt
1 teaspoon black
   peppercorns
3 bay leaves
10 cups water

Homemade chicken stock is always useful in the kitchen, so I like to have several quart containers in the freezer at all times. Make a Whole Chicken (page 104), then cut off all the meat and use the carcass (wings, neck, backs, leftover carcass) to make this delicious, simple chicken stock.

---

1. In the Instant Pot, combine the chicken bones, onion, carrots, celery, garlic, salt, peppercorns, and bay leaves.

2. Add the water, making sure not to go past the "max fill" line. Secure the lid and cook on high pressure for 1 hour.

3. After cooking, let the pressure release naturally for 30 minutes, then quick release the remaining pressure. Unlock and remove the lid, then mix well.

4. Strain the stock through a fine-mesh strainer or colander into a large bowl. Discard the solids, and cool the stock for 30 minutes.

SAVE FOR LATER: Portion out chicken stock into airtight containers, and store in the refrigerator for up to 1 week or in the freezer for up to 3 months. If freezing, you can portion out stock into resealable freezer bags and place several in a stack flat on a baking sheet. Once frozen, remove the baking sheet, and keep the frozen stock stacked in the freezer.

BASIL-WALNUT PESTO

GLUTEN-FREE
Makes 1 cup
Prep time: 10 minutes
Total time: 10 minutes

PER SERVING
(2 TABLESPOONS): Calories:
175; Fat: 18g; Carbohydrates:
2g; Fiber: 1g;
Sugar: 0g; Protein: 4g;
Sodium: 175mg

---

2 cups loosely packed
fresh basil leaves
⅓ cup chopped
walnuts
⅓ cup grated
Parmesan cheese
1 garlic clove, peeled
½ teaspoon kosher salt
¼ teaspoon freshly
ground black pepper
⅓ cup extra-virgin
olive oil

Pesto is one of my go-to secrets when I need to add a pop of flavor to a dish. This version is slightly different than a classic version, with walnuts taking the place of pine nuts. You can easily adjust the recipe to include whatever herbs and nuts you have on hand. For a spicy kick, add a pinch of red pepper flakes! This versatile pesto tastes great paired with pasta, fish, meat, poultry, and roasted vegetables.

---

1. In a food processor, combine the basil, walnuts, cheese, garlic, salt, and pepper. Pulse 8 to 10 times.

2. Continue to process while adding the oil until your desired consistency is reached.

SAVE FOR LATER: Freeze any leftover pesto in ice cube trays. Simply pop out the pesto cubes once they're frozen, and store in a resealable freezer bag. You'll be able to grab a perfectly portioned pesto cube any time and add it to your favorite meals!

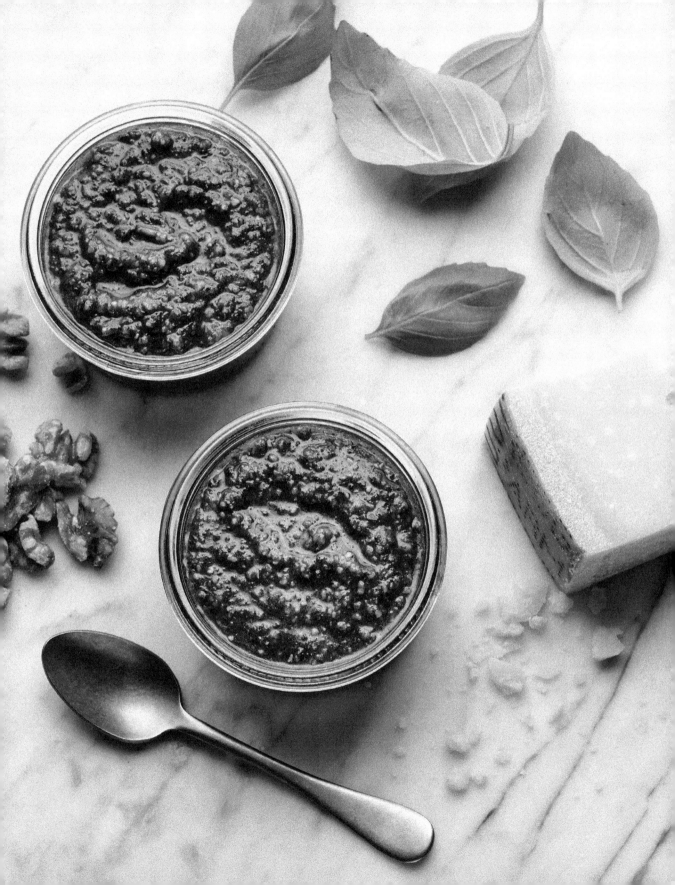

TAHINI DRESSING

**DAIRY-FREE,
GLUTEN-FREE**

Makes 2 cups
Prep time: 10 minutes
Total time: 10 minutes

PER SERVING
(2 TABLESPOONS): Calories:
165; Fat: 18g; Carbohydrates:
2g; Fiber: 1g;
Sugar: 0g; Protein: 1g;
Sodium: 310mg

SIMPLE SWAP: Tamari
is gluten-free soy sauce,
but if you are not following a gluten-free diet, feel
free to use low-sodium
soy sauce in its place.

This delightful Tahini Dressing goes well as a salad dressing; can be drizzled over roasted vegetables, meat, or poultry; and can even be used as a dip-ping sauce. It stays fresh in the refrigerator for up to 2 weeks. Simply remove from the refrigerator a few minutes before serving to allow it to come to room temperature, then shake or whisk well.

1 cup extra-virgin olive oil
½ cup water
⅓ cup tahini
¼ cup tamari
¼ cup freshly squeezed lemon juice
2 tablespoons sesame oil
1½ teaspoons dry mustard
¾ teaspoon kosher salt
⅛ teaspoon cayenne pepper

In a medium bowl, whisk together the olive oil, water, tahini, tamari, lemon juice, sesame oil, mustard, salt, and cayenne. (You can also use an immersion blender.)

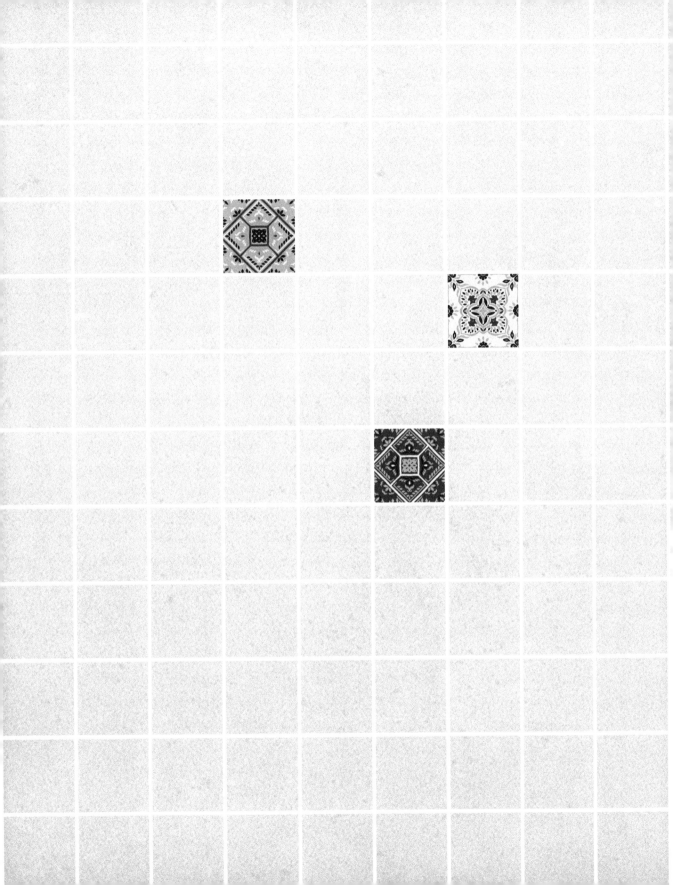

INSTANT POT COOKING CHARTS

These charts are intended to be used as helpful cooking aids for those looking to do more in the kitchen with their Instant Pot and have been included as a resourceful guide to cooking the basics, not just the recipes in this book.

Beans and Legumes

Although the recipes in this book call for unsoaked beans, for those interested in cooking soaked beans in their Instant Pot, the cooking times below are for beans that have been soaked for 8 to 24 hours in salted water, unless otherwise noted.

	Minutes Under Pressure	Pressure	Release
Black beans	10	High	Natural for 15 to 20 minutes, then quick
Black-eyed peas	10	High	Natural for 15 to 20 minutes, then quick
Cannellini beans	5	High	Natural for 15 to 20 minutes, then quick
Chickpeas (garbanzo beans)	20	High	Natural for 15 to 20 minutes, then quick
Kidney beans	20	High	Natural for 15 to 20 minutes, then quick
Brown lentils (unsoaked)	20	High	Natural for 15 to 20 minutes, then quick
Red lentils (unsoaked)	10	High	Natural for 10 minutes, then quick
Pinto beans	20	High	Natural for 5 minutes, then quick
Split peas (unsoaked)	10	High	Natural for 15 to 20 minutes, then quick
Lima beans	15	High	Natural for 15 to 20 minutes, then quick
Soybeans, dried	15	High	Natural for 15 to 20 minutes, then quick
Soybeans, fresh (edamame), unsoaked	1	High	Quick

Grains

To prevent foaming, rinse grains thoroughly before cooking.

	Liquid per 1 cup of grain	Minutes Under Pressure	Pressure	Release
Arborio rice (for risotto)	3 to 4 cups	6 to 8	High	Natural for 15 minutes, then quick
Barley, pearled	2½ cups	20	High	Natural for 10 minutes, then quick
Brown rice, medium-grain	1 cup	15	Low	Natural for 15 to 20 minutes, then quick
Brown rice, long-grain	1 cup	15	Low	Natural for 20 minutes, then quick
Buckwheat	1¾ cups	12 to 15	High	Natural for 15 to 20 minutes, then quick
Farro, pearled	2 cups	6 to 8	High	Natural for 15 to 20 minutes, then quick
Farro, whole-grain	3 cups	22 to 25	High	Natural for 15 to 20 minutes, then quick
Oats, rolled	3 cups	3 to 4	High	Quick
Oats, steel-cut	3 cups	10	High	Natural for 10 minutes, then quick
Quinoa	1½ cups	8	High	Natural for 15 minutes, then Quick
Wheat berries	2 cups	30	High	Natural for 10 minutes, then quick
White rice, long-grain	1 cup	5 to 8	High	Natural for 15 to 20 minutes, then quick
Wild rice	1¼ cups	22 to 25	High	Natural for 15 to 20 minutes, then quick

Meat

Except as noted, these times are for braised meats—that is, meats that are seared before pressure cooking and partially submerged in liquid.

	Minutes Under Pressure	Pressure	Release
Beef, bone-in short ribs	30 to 40	High	Natural for 30 to 40 minutes, then quick
Beef, flat iron steak, cut into ½-inch strips	6	Low	Quick
Beef, shoulder (chuck) roast (2 pounds)	35 to 45	High	Natural for 30 to 40 minutes, then quick
Beef, shoulder (chuck), 2-inch chunks	20	High	Natural for 10 minutes, then quick
Beef, sirloin steak, cut into ½-inch strips	3	Low	Quick
Lamb, shanks	45	High	Natural for 30 to 40 minutes, then quick
Lamb, shoulder, 2-inch chunks	35	High	Natural for 30 to 40 minutes, then quick
Pork, back ribs (steamed)	25	High	Quick
Pork, shoulder roast (2 pounds)	25	High	Natural for 30 to 40 minutes, then quick
Pork, shoulder, 2-inch chunks	20	High	Quick
Pork, spare ribs (steamed)	20	High	Quick
Pork, tenderloin	4	Low	Quick
Smoked pork sausage, ½-inch slices	5 to 10	High	Quick

Poultry

Except as noted, these times are for braised poultry—that is, partially submerged in liquid.

	Minutes Under Pressure	Pressure	Release
Chicken breast, bone-in	15	High	Quick
Chicken breast, boneless	5 (steamed)	Low	Natural for 8 minutes, then quick
Chicken thigh, bone-in	15 to 25	High	Natural for 20 minutes, then quick
Chicken thigh, boneless	15 to 25	High	Natural for 20 minutes, then quick
Chicken, whole	20 to 30	High	Natural for 15 minutes, then quick
Duck quarters, bone-in	35	High	Quick
Turkey breast, tenderloin, 12 ounces	5 (steamed)	Low	Natural for 8 minutes, then quick
Turkey thigh, bone-in	30	High	Natural for 20 minutes, then quick

Fish and Seafood

All times are for steamed fish and shellfish.

	Minutes Under Pressure	Pressure	Release
Clams	4	High	Natural for 15 minutes, then quick
Halibut (1-inch thick)	3	High	Quick
Mussels	2	High	Quick
Salmon (1-inch thick)	3	Low	Quick
Shrimp, large (frozen)	1	Low	Quick
Tilapia or cod	3	Low	Quick

Vegetables

The cooking method for all the following vegetables is steaming; if the vegetables are cooked in liquid, the times may vary. Green vegetables will be tender-crisp; root vegetables will be soft.

	Prep	Minutes Under Pressure	Pressure	Release
Acorn squash	Halved	9	High	Quick
Artichokes, large	Whole	8	High	Quick
Beets	Whole	20	High	Quick
Broccoli	Cut into florets	0 to 1	Low	Quick
Brussels sprouts	Halved	2	High	Quick
Butternut squash	Peeled, cut into ½-inch chunks	8	High	Quick
Cabbage	Sliced	3 to 4	High	Quick
Carrots	½- to 1-inch slices	2	High	Quick
Cauliflower	Whole	6	High	Quick
Cauliflower	Cut into florets	0 to 1	Low	Quick
Green beans	Cut in half or thirds	0 to 3	Low	Quick
Potatoes, large russet	Quartered; for mashing	8	High	Natural for 8 minutes, then quick
Potatoes, red	Whole if less than 1½ inch across, halved if larger	4	High	Quick
Spaghetti squash	Halved lengthwise	7	High	Quick
Sweet potatoes	Halved lengthwise	12	High	Quick

MEASUREMENT CONVERSIONS

VOLUME EQUIVALENTS	U.S. STANDARD	U.S. STANDARD (OUNCES)	METRIC (APPROXIMATE)
LIQUID	2 tablespoons	1 fl. oz.	30 mL
	¼ cup	2 fl. oz.	60 mL
	½ cup	4 fl. oz.	120 mL
	1 cup	8 fl. oz.	240 mL
	1½ cups	12 fl. oz.	355 mL
	2 cups or 1 pint	16 fl. oz.	475 mL
	4 cups or 1 quart	32 fl. oz.	1 L
	1 gallon	128 fl. oz.	4 L
DRY	⅛ teaspoon		0.5 mL
	¼ teaspoon		1 mL
	½ teaspoon		2 mL
	¾ teaspoon		4 mL
	1 teaspoon		5 mL
	1 tablespoon		15 mL
	¼ cup		59 mL
	⅓ cup		79 mL
	½ cup		118 mL
	⅔ cup		156 mL
	¾ cup		177 mL
	1 cup		235 mL
	2 cups or 1 pint		475 mL
	3 cups		700 mL
	4 cups or 1 quart		1 L
	½ gallon		2 L
	1 gallon		4 L

OVEN TEMPERATURES

FAHRENHEIT	CELSIUS (APPROXIMATE)
250°F	120°C
300°F	150°C
325°F	165°C
350°F	180°C
375°F	190°C
400°F	200°C
425°F	220°C
450°F	230°C

WEIGHT EQUIVALENTS

U.S. STANDARD	METRIC (APPROXIMATE)
½ ounce	15 g
1 ounce	30 g
2 ounces	60 g
4 ounces	115 g
8 ounces	225 g
12 ounces	340 g
16 ounces or 1 pound	455 g

REFERENCE

Yu, Zhi, Vasanti S. Malik, NaNa Keum, Frank B. Hu, Edward L. Giovannucci, Meir J. Stampfer, Walter C. Willett, et al. "Associations Between Nut Consumption and Inflammatory Biomarkers." *The American Journal of Clinical Nutrition, Volume* 104, Issue 3 (September 2016): pages 722–28. doi.org/10.3945/ajcn.116.134205.

INDEX

A

Almond Butter Oatmeal, 24
Apples, Baked, 120
Artichokes with Yogurt Aïoli, 36
Asparagus
  Green Chicken Soup, 105
  Risotto with Mushrooms and
      Asparagus, 64–65
Avgolemono (Greek Chicken
    and Egg Soup), 95
Avocado, Egg Salad with, 32

B

Basil
  Basil-Walnut Pesto, 142
  Salmon with Basil-Walnut Pesto, 90
  Spaghetti Squash with Cherry
      Tomatoes, Basil, and Feta, 67
Beans, 14–15
  Basic Beans, 135
  Bean Salad, 44
  Bean Soup, 52
  cooking chart, 146
  Monkfish with Kale and
      White Beans, 86–87
  Sausage-Bean Soup, 94
  Smashed Fava Beans with
      Toast, 43
Beef, 17
  cooking chart, 148
  Mediterranean-Style Brisket, 100–101
Beets with Tahini Yogurt, 39
Berry Compote with Yogurt, 121
Branzino, Whole, 91

Burgers, Red Lentil, 58–59
Butternut Squash and Chickpeas,
    Moroccan Tagine with, 61–62

C

Cabbage, Deconstructed
    Lamb-Stuffed, 107
Cardamom, Poached Pears with, 122
Chicken, 16
  Avgolemono (Greek Chicken
      and Egg Soup), 95
  Braised Chicken with Tomato
      and Olives, 111–112
  Chicken Stock, 141
  Chicken with Mushrooms, 113
  Chicken with Peppers, 116–117
  cooking chart, 149
  Green Chicken Soup, 105
  Lemon Chicken with Rosemary, 106
  Shredded Chicken with Harissa, 99
  Whole Chicken, 104
Chickpeas
  Hummus, 138
  Moroccan Tagine with Butternut
      Squash and Chickpeas, 61–62
  Spiced Chickpea Bowls, 63
Chile Sauce, Halibut with Tomato-, 82–83
Chocolate Pots de Crème, 124–125
Chraimeh Sauce, Green Beans with, 38
Clams, Steamed, 89
Cod with Puttanesca, 88
Couscous with Eggplant, 72
Crème Fraîche, Creamy Polenta with, 42

Cucumbers
  Tzatziki, 139
Custard with Roasted Fruit, 128–129

D

Dairy-free
  Almond Butter Oatmeal, 24
  Avgolemono (Greek Chicken
    and Egg Soup), 95
  Baked Apples, 120
  Basic Beans, 135
  Basic Brown Rice, 134
  Bean Salad, 44
  Bean Soup, 52
  Braised Chicken with Tomato
    and Olives, 111–112
  Chicken Stock, 141
  Chicken with Mushrooms, 113
  Chicken with Peppers, 116–117
  Cod with Puttanesca, 88
  Cold-Poached Salmon Salad, 78
  Couscous with Eggplant, 72
  Deconstructed Lamb-
    Stuffed Cabbage, 107
  Eggplant, Summer Squash,
    and Tomatoes, 37
  Egg Salad with Avocado, 32
  Greek-Style Lentils, 46–47
  Green Beans with Chraimeh Sauce, 38
  Green Chicken Soup, 105
  Halibut with Tomato-Chile
    Sauce, 82–83
  Hard- and Soft-Boiled Eggs, 136
  Hummus, 138
  Jammy Eggs with Hummus
    and Rice Salad, 69

Lemon Chicken with Rosemary, 106
Mediterranean-Style Brisket, 100–101
Monkfish with Kale and
  White Beans, 86–87
Moroccan Lamb, 102–103
Moroccan Tagine with Butternut
  Squash and Chickpeas, 61–62
Mussels with Harissa, 76
Osso Buco, 97–98
Poached Pears with Cardamom, 122
Poached Shrimp with Mediterranean
  "Cocktail Sauce," 85
Pork Ragù, 114–115
Potatoes with Greens, 40
Red Lentil Burgers, 58–59
Sausage-Bean Soup, 94
Shredded Chicken with Harissa, 99
Shrimp with Lentils, 80–81
Smashed Potatoes, 41
Steamed Clams, 89
Tahini Dressing, 144
Tuna Niçoise Salad, 79
Vegetable Stock, 140
Whole Branzino, 91
Whole Chicken, 104
Dairy products, 17
Desserts
  Baked Apples, 120
  Berry Compote with Yogurt, 121
  Chocolate Pots de Crème, 124–125
  Custard with Roasted Fruit, 128–129
  Nut and Fig "Pudding" with
    Yogurt Cream, 126–127
  Poached Pears with Cardamom, 122
  Rice Pudding, 130–131

Dressing, Tahini, 144
Duck, 16, 149

E

Eggplants
  Couscous with Eggplant, 72
  Eggplant, Summer Squash,
    and Tomatoes, 37
  Lentil and Eggplant Stew, 53
Eggs, 16–17
  Avgolemono (Greek Chicken
    and Egg Soup), 95
  Coddled Eggs with Spinach, 31
  Egg Bites, 25
  Egg Salad with Avocado, 32
  Hard- and Soft-Boiled Eggs, 136
  Jammy Eggs with Hummus
    and Rice Salad, 69
  Savory Strata, 28–29
  Zucchini Frittata, 30

F

Farro with Herby Yogurt, 48
Fava Beans with Toast, Smashed, 43
Feta, Spaghetti Squash with Cherry
    Tomatoes, Basil, and, 67
Fig "Pudding" with Yogurt Cream,
    Nut and, 126–127
Fish and seafood, 16, 18
  Cod with Puttanesca, 88
  Cold-Poached Salmon Salad, 78
  cooking chart, 150
  Halibut with Tomato-Chile
    Sauce, 82–83
  Monkfish with Kale and
    White Beans, 86–87

Mussels with Harissa, 76
Poached Shrimp with Mediterranean
    "Cocktail Sauce," 85
Salmon with Basil-Walnut Pesto, 90
Shrimp with Lentils, 80–81
Steamed Clams, 89
Tuna Niçoise Salad, 79
Whole Branzino, 91
Fruits, 14. *See also specific*
  Custard with Roasted Fruit, 128–129

G

Gluten-free
  Almond Butter Oatmeal, 24
  Artichokes with Yogurt Aïoli, 36
  Avgolemono (Greek Chicken
    and Egg Soup), 95
  Baked Apples, 120
  Basic Beans, 135
  Basic Brown Rice, 134
  Basil-Walnut Pesto, 142
  Bean Salad, 44
  Bean Soup, 52
  Beets with Tahini Yogurt, 39
  Berry Compote with Yogurt, 121
  Braised Chicken with Tomato
    and Olives, 111–112
  Chicken Stock, 141
  Chicken with Mushrooms, 113
  Chicken with Peppers, 116–117
  Chocolate Pots de Crème, 124–125
  Coddled Eggs with Spinach, 31
  Cod with Puttanesca, 88
  Cold-Poached Salmon Salad, 78
  Creamy Polenta with
    Crème Fraîche, 42

Custard with Roasted Fruit, 128–129
Deconstructed Lamb-
    Stuffed Cabbage, 107
Egg Bites, 25
Eggplant, Summer Squash,
    and Tomatoes, 37
Greek-Style Lentils, 46–47
Green Beans with Chraimeh
    Sauce, 38
Halibut with Tomato-Chile
    Sauce, 82–83
Hard- and Soft-Boiled Eggs, 136
Hummus, 138
Jammy Eggs with Hummus
    and Rice Salad, 69
Lemon Chicken with Rosemary, 106
Lentil and Eggplant Stew, 53
Lentil Ragù, 70–71
Mediterranean-Style Brisket, 100–101
Monkfish with Kale and
    White Beans, 86–87
Gluten-free (continued)
Moroccan Lamb, 102–103
Moroccan Tagine with Butternut
    Squash and Chickpeas, 61–62
Mujadara, 54–55
Mussels with Harissa, 76
Nut and Fig "Pudding" with
    Yogurt Cream, 126–127
Plain Yogurt, 137
Poached Pears with
    Cardamom, 122
Poached Shrimp with Mediterranean
    "Cocktail Sauce," 85
Pork Ragù, 114–115
Potatoes with Greens, 40

Red Lentil Burgers, 58–59
Rice Pudding, 130–131
Risotto with Mushrooms and
    Asparagus, 64–65
Salmon with Basil-Walnut Pesto, 90
Sausage-Bean Soup, 94
Shredded Chicken with Harissa, 99
Shrimp with Lentils, 80–81
Smashed Potatoes, 41
Spaghetti Squash with Cherry
    Tomatoes, Basil, and Feta, 67
Spiced Chickpea Bowls, 63
Steamed Clams, 89
Stuffed Sweet Potatoes, 66
Tahini Dressing, 144
Tuna Niçoise Salad, 79
Tzatziki, 139
Vegetable Stock, 140
Whole Branzino, 91
Whole Chicken, 104
Yogurt Parfait, 26
Zucchini Frittata, 30
Grains, 15, 147
Green Beans with Chraimeh Sauce, 38
Greens, Potatoes with, 40

H

Halibut with Tomato-Chile
    Sauce, 82–83
Harissa, 19
  Mussels with Harissa, 76
  Shredded Chicken with
    Harissa, 99
Herbs, 19
High altitude cooking, 11
Hummus, 138

Jammy Eggs with Hummus
and Rice Salad, 69

I

Instant Pots
accessories, 7–8
benefits of, 3
cleaning, 9
cooking charts, 146–151
how they work, 3–4
safety, 6–7
settings, 5–6
troubleshooting, 10–11

K

Kale and White Beans
Monkfish with, 86–87

L

Lamb, 17
cooking chart, 148
Deconstructed Lamb-
Stuffed Cabbage, 107
Lamb Meat Loaf with Tahini
Sauce, 108–109
Moroccan Lamb, 102–103
Legumes, 14–15, 146
Lemon Chicken with Rosemary, 106
Lentils
Greek-Style Lentils, 46–47
Lentil and Eggplant Stew, 53
Lentil Ragù, 70–71
Mujadara, 54–55
Red Lentil Burgers, 58–59
Shrimp with Lentils, 80–81

M

Meats, 17, 148. *See also specific*
Mediterranean diet, 1–2, 13
Mediterranean region, 4
Monkfish with Kale and White
Beans, 86–87
Mujadara, 54–55
Mushrooms
Chicken with Mushrooms, 113
Risotto with Mushrooms and
Asparagus, 64–65
Mussels with Harissa, 76

N

Nuts, 19
Basil-Walnut Pesto, 142
Nut and Fig "Pudding" with
Yogurt Cream, 126–127
Salmon with Basil-Walnut
Pesto, 90

O

Oatmeal, Almond Butter, 24
Oils, 18–19
Olives, Braised Chicken with
Tomato and, 111–112
Osso Buco, 97–98

P

Pasta with Marinara Sauce, 68
Pears with Cardamom, Poached, 122
Peppers, Chicken with, 116–117
Pesto
Basil-Walnut Pesto, 142
Salmon with Basil-Walnut Pesto, 90
Physical activity, 2

Polenta with Crème Fraîche,
    Creamy, 42
Pork, 17
    cooking chart, 148
    Pork Ragù, 114–115
Potatoes
    Potatoes with Greens, 40
    Smashed Potatoes, 41
Poultry, 16, 149
Pressure cooking, 4
Puttanesca, Cod with, 88

R

Ragù
    Lentil Ragù, 70–71
    Pork Ragù, 114–115
Recipes, about, 20–21
Releasing pressure, 6, 7
Rice
    Basic Brown Rice, 134
    Jammy Eggs with Hummus
        and Rice Salad, 69
    Mujadara, 54–55
    Rice Pudding, 130–131
    Risotto with Mushrooms and
        Asparagus, 64–65
Rosemary, Lemon Chicken
    with, 106

S

Safety tips, 6–7
Salads
    Bean Salad, 44
    Cold-Poached Salmon
        Salad, 78
    Egg Salad with Avocado, 32

Jammy Eggs with Hummus
    and Rice Salad, 69
Tuna Niçoise Salad, 79
Salmon
    Cold-Poached Salmon Salad, 78
    cooking chart, 150
    Salmon with Basil-Walnut
        Pesto, 90
Sausage-Bean Soup, 94
Seeds, 19
Shrimp
    cooking chart, 150
    Poached Shrimp with Mediterranean
        "Cocktail Sauce," 85
    Shrimp with Lentils, 80–81
Soups and stews
    Avgolemono (Greek Chicken
        and Egg Soup), 95
    Bean Soup, 52
    Green Chicken Soup, 105
    Lentil and Eggplant Stew, 53
    Moroccan Tagine with Butternut
        Squash and Chickpeas, 61–62
    Sausage-Bean Soup, 94
    Vegetable Bourguignon, 56–57
Spaghetti Squash with Cherry
    Tomatoes, Basil, and Feta, 67
Spices, 19
Spinach, Coddled Eggs with, 31
Squash
    Eggplant, Summer Squash,
        and Tomatoes, 37
    Moroccan Tagine with Butternut
        Squash and Chickpeas, 61–62
    Spaghetti Squash with Cherry
        Tomatoes, Basil, and Feta, 67

Zucchini Frittata, 30
Stocks
  Chicken Stock, 141
  Vegetable Stock, 140
Sugar, 20
Sumac, 19
Sweet Potatoes, Stuffed, 66

T

Tagine with Butternut Squash and
    Chickpeas, Moroccan, 61–62
Tahini
  Beets with Tahini Yogurt, 39
  Hummus, 138
  Lamb Meat Loaf with Tahini
    Sauce, 108–109
  Tahini Dressing, 144
Toast, Smashed Fava Beans with, 43
Tomatoes
  Braised Chicken with Tomato
    and Olives, 111–112
  Eggplant, Summer Squash,
    and Tomatoes, 37
  Halibut with Tomato-Chile
    Sauce, 82–83
  Pasta with Marinara Sauce, 68
  Spaghetti Squash with Cherry
    Tomatoes, Basil, and Feta, 67
Troubleshooting, 10–11
Tuna Niçoise Salad, 79
Turkey, 16, 149
Tzatziki, 139

V

Veal
  Osso Buco, 97–98

Vegetables, 14. *See also specific*
  cooking chart, 151
  starchy, 15
  Vegetable Bourguignon, 56–57
  Vegetable Stock, 140

W

Walnuts
  Basil-Walnut Pesto, 142
  Salmon with Basil-Walnut
    Pesto, 90
Wine, 20

Y

Yogurt
  Artichokes with Yogurt Aïoli, 36
  Beets with Tahini Yogurt, 39
  Berry Compote with Yogurt, 121
  Farro with Herby Yogurt, 48
  Nut and Fig "Pudding" with
    Yogurt Cream, 126–127
  Plain Yogurt, 137
  Tzatziki, 139
  Yogurt Parfait, 26

Z

Za'atar, 19
Zucchini Frittata, 30

ABOUT THE AUTHOR

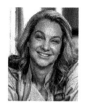 Chef **Abbie Gellman**, MS, RD, CDN, is a spokesperson, recipe and product developer, educator, and nationally recognized culinary nutrition expert. She creates, produces, and hosts cooking and nutrition videos and works with a wide variety of food companies/brands, commodity boards, food service operators, health professionals, and private clients. She is regularly featured in the media and contributes to many publications as both an expert and an author. Her first cookbook, *The Mediterranean DASH Diet*, was published November 2019. She is the consulting "Better for You" R&D Chef/RD for the private company Happi Foodi and has created two lines of healthy frozen meals for them under the Walmart Better For You Great Value brand and the Happi Foodi brand; both can currently be found at Walmart. Abbie lives i n NYC with her daughter, Olivia, and many shelves of cookbooks. Learn more about her at ChefAbbieGellman.com and connect with her via @ChefAbbieGellman on Instagram, YouTube, Facebook, and Pinterest.

CPSIA information can be obtained
at www.ICGtesting.com
Printed in the USA
JSHW010230250422
25239JS00001B/1